I Love Yoga

Anita Raina Thapan

Illustrated by Alankrita

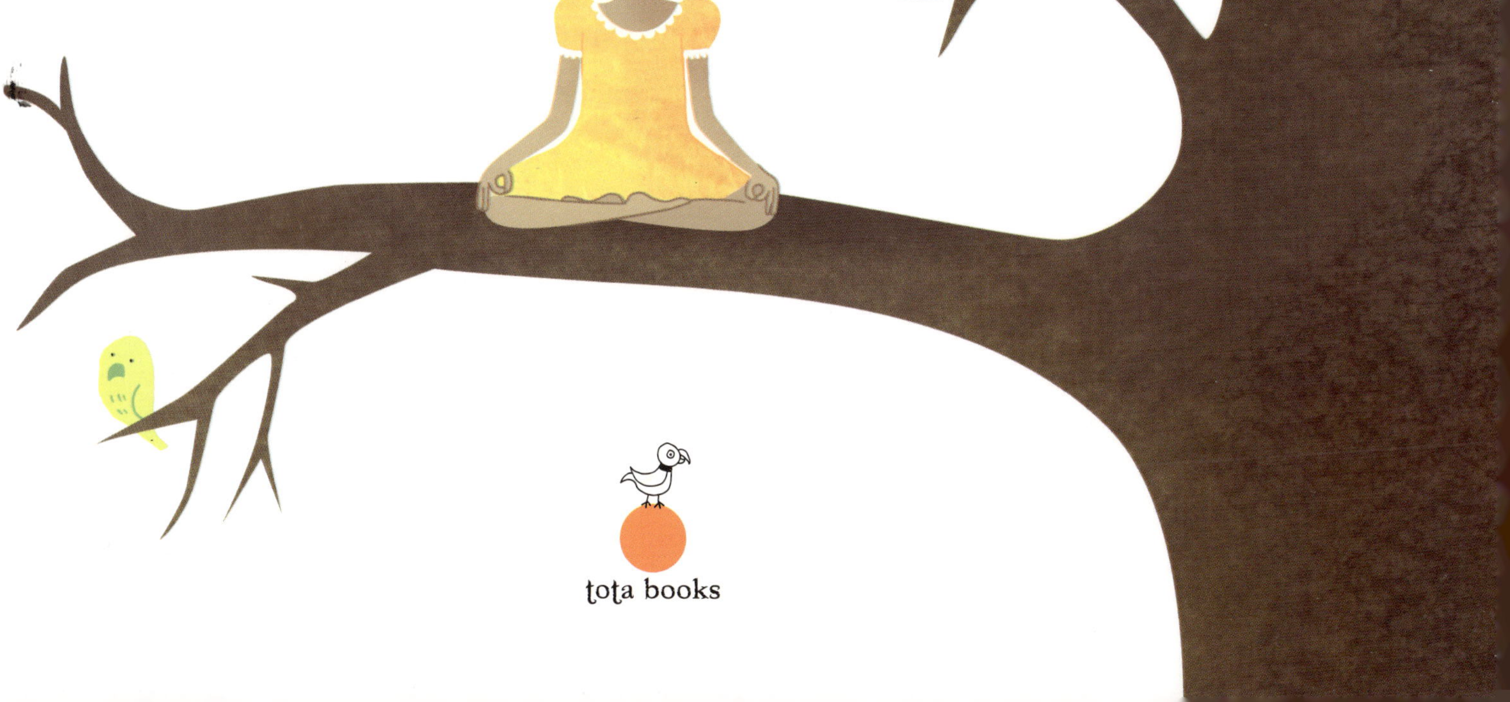

tota books

tota books

I LOVE YOGA

Illustrations by Alankrita

First Indian Paperback Edition, 2016
First Reprint, 2017
Second Reprint, 2020
Third Reprint, 2023

ISBN 978-81-7621-290-8

Published by tota books
J-40, Jorbagh Lane, New Delhi-110003
Tel: 011-24621011
contact@fullcirclebooks.in • www.fullcirclebooks.in

Printed at Ask Advertising Aids Private Limited, New Delhi-110020 India

PRINTED IN INDIA

For Tarak and Avani,
whose enthusiasm for yoga is unforgettable!

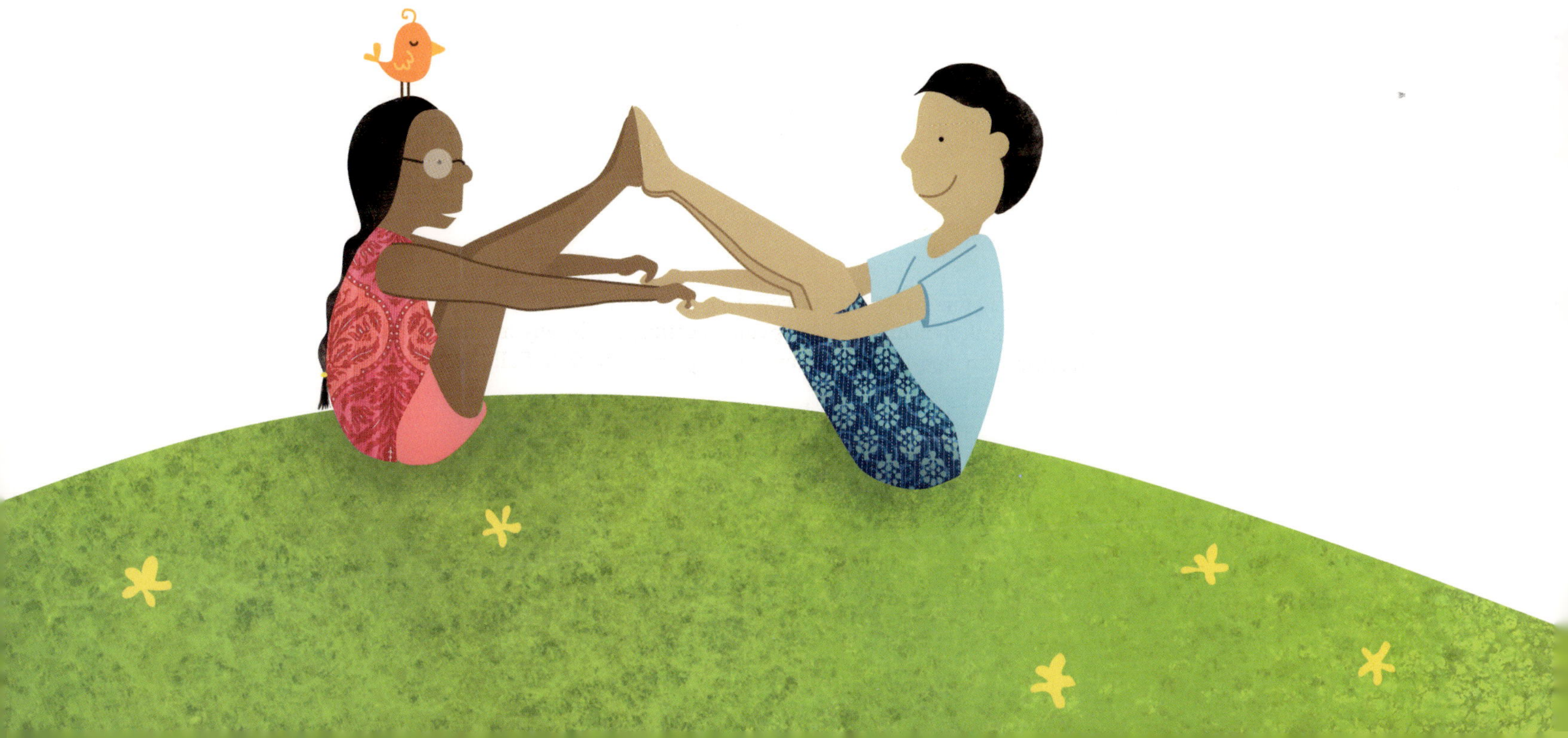

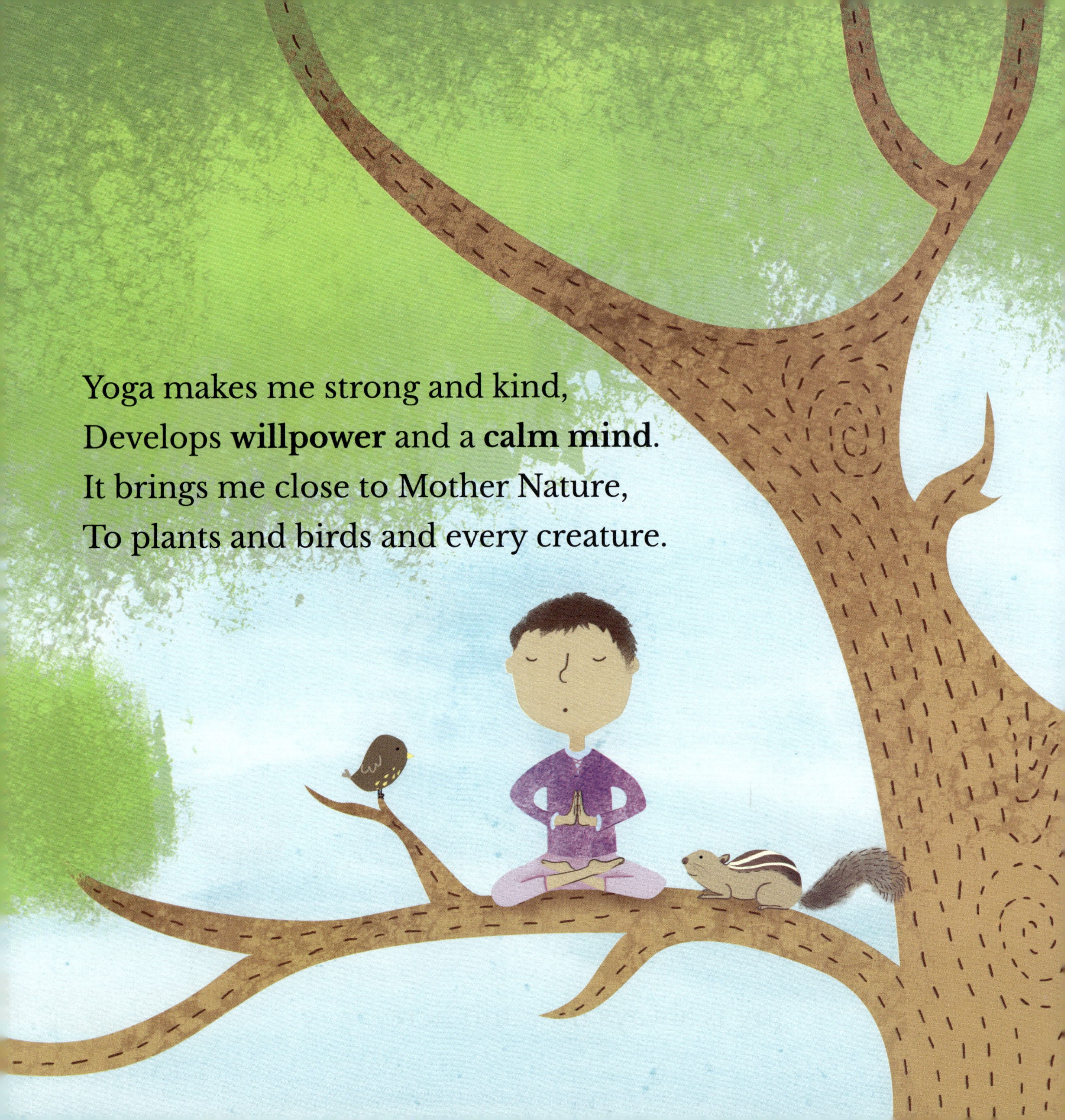

Yoga makes me strong and kind,
Develops **willpower** and a **calm mind**.
It brings me close to Mother Nature,
To plants and birds and every creature.

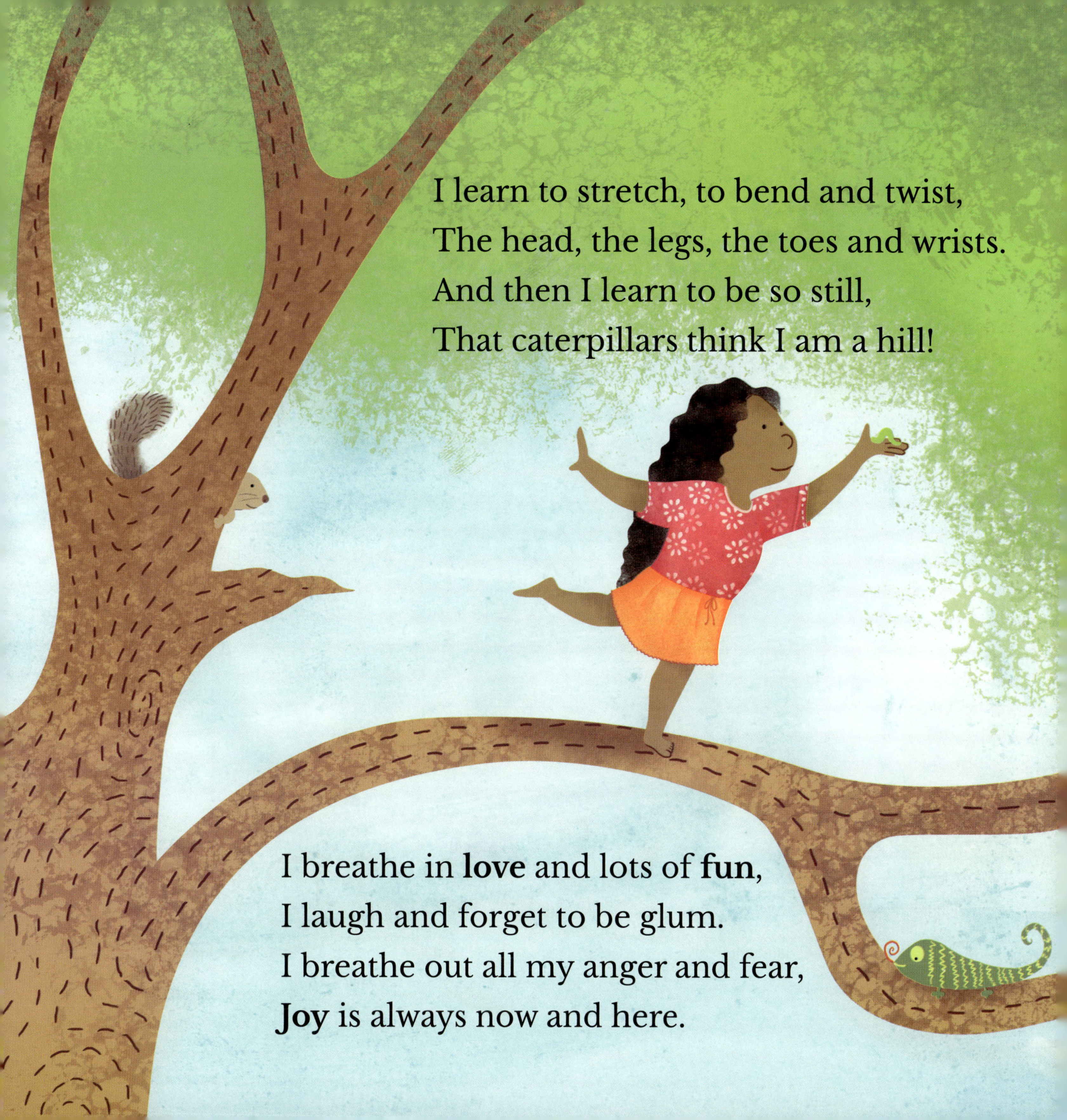

I learn to stretch, to bend and twist,
The head, the legs, the toes and wrists.
And then I learn to be so still,
That caterpillars think I am a hill!

I breathe in **love** and lots of **fun**,
I laugh and forget to be glum.
I breathe out all my anger and fear,
Joy is always now and here.

Shavasana - Corpse Pose

I lie down and close my eyes,
my back feels good against the ground.
I am still, there is no sound.

Then I stretch my hands and toes,
Turning to the side, I raise myself.
And sit up straight,
With crossed legs.

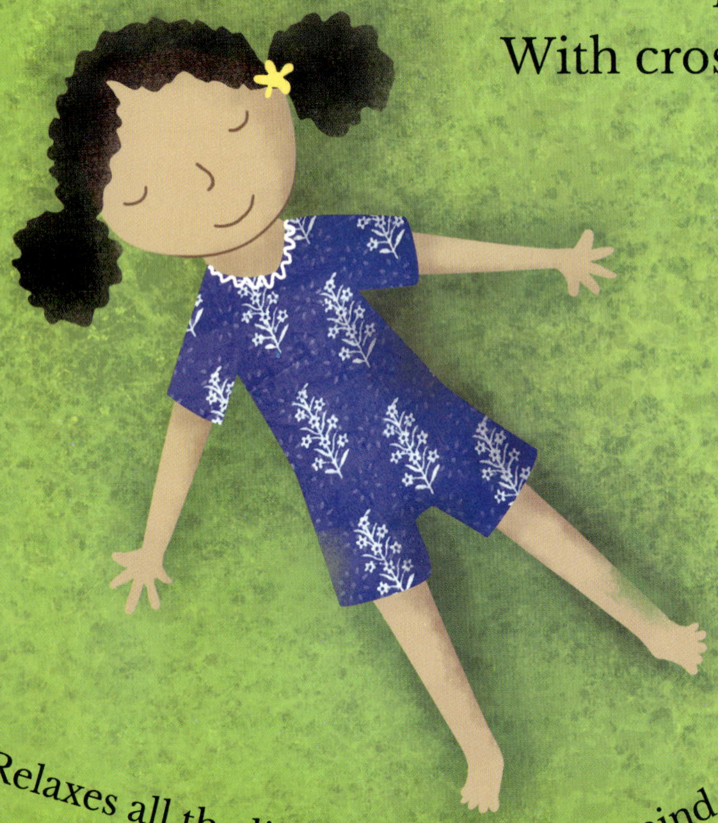

Relaxes all the limbs, joints and the mind, breath becomes slow and steady.

Prayer

Om! Om! Om! Thank you, Shiva,
Thank you, all the teachers of yoga.
Because of you, I can learn today,
How to be better in every way.

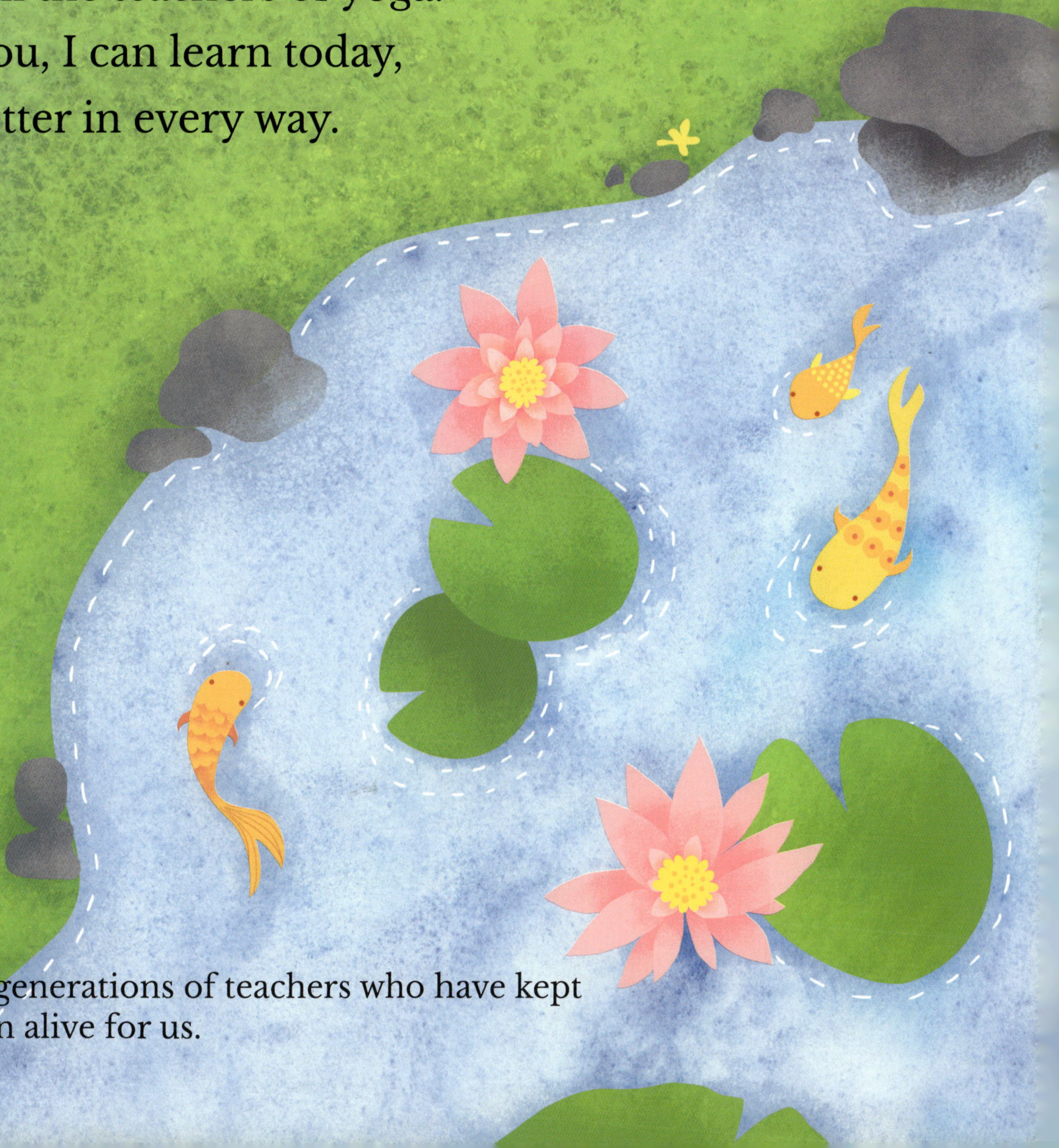

Gratitude to all the generations of teachers who have kept this ancient tradition alive for us.

Vrikshasana - Dynamic Tree Pose

I am a little seed in the ground,
Slowly I grow and become a tree.
My arms are branches spread around,
My legs the trunk, my fingers the leaves.

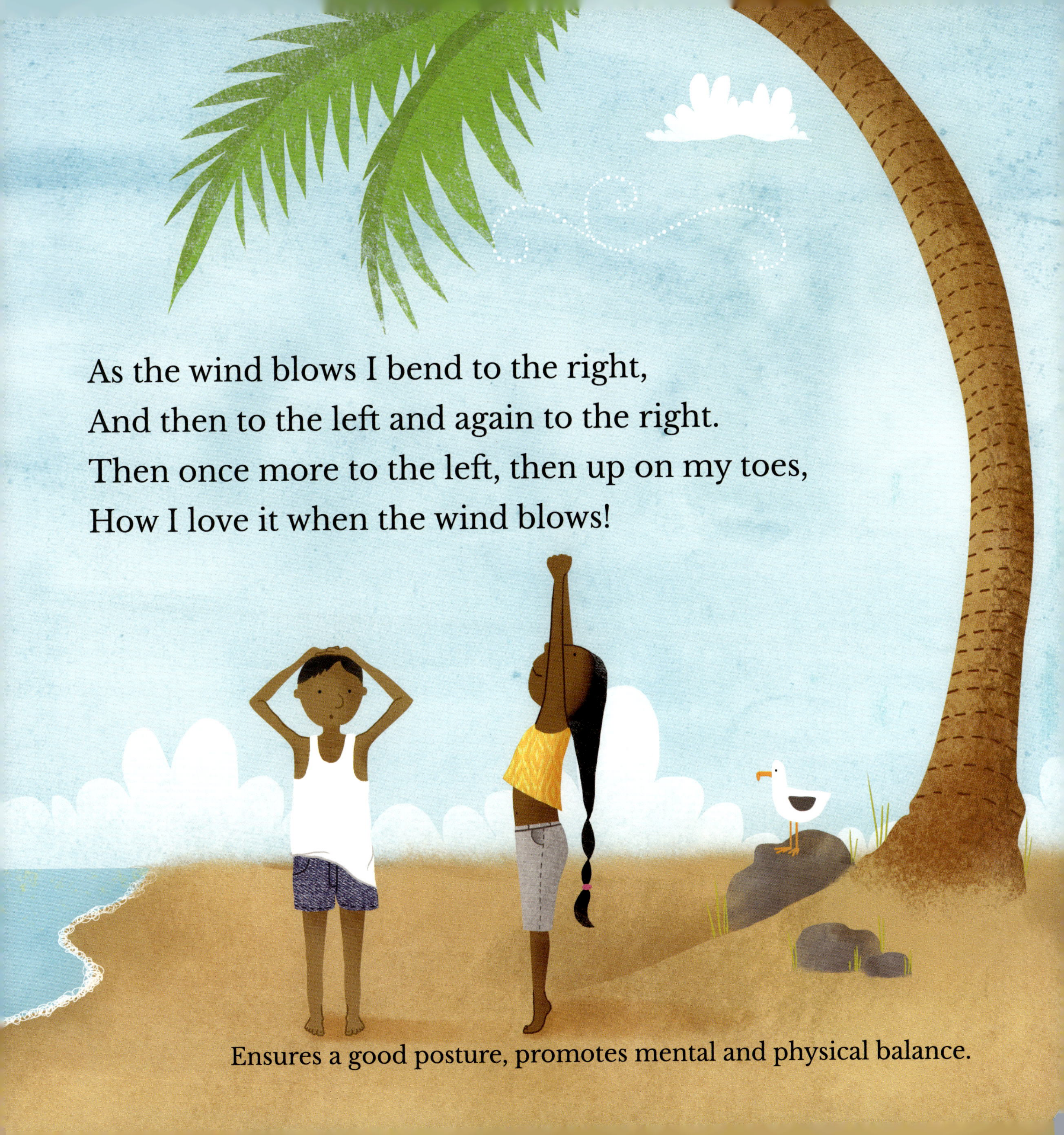

As the wind blows I bend to the right,
And then to the left and again to the right.
Then once more to the left, then up on my toes,
How I love it when the wind blows!

Ensures a good posture, promotes mental and physical balance.

Parvatasana - Mountain Pose

I bend and place my hands on the ground,
My body becomes a mountain high.
I imagine there is snow all around,
I breathe in and out for a count of five.

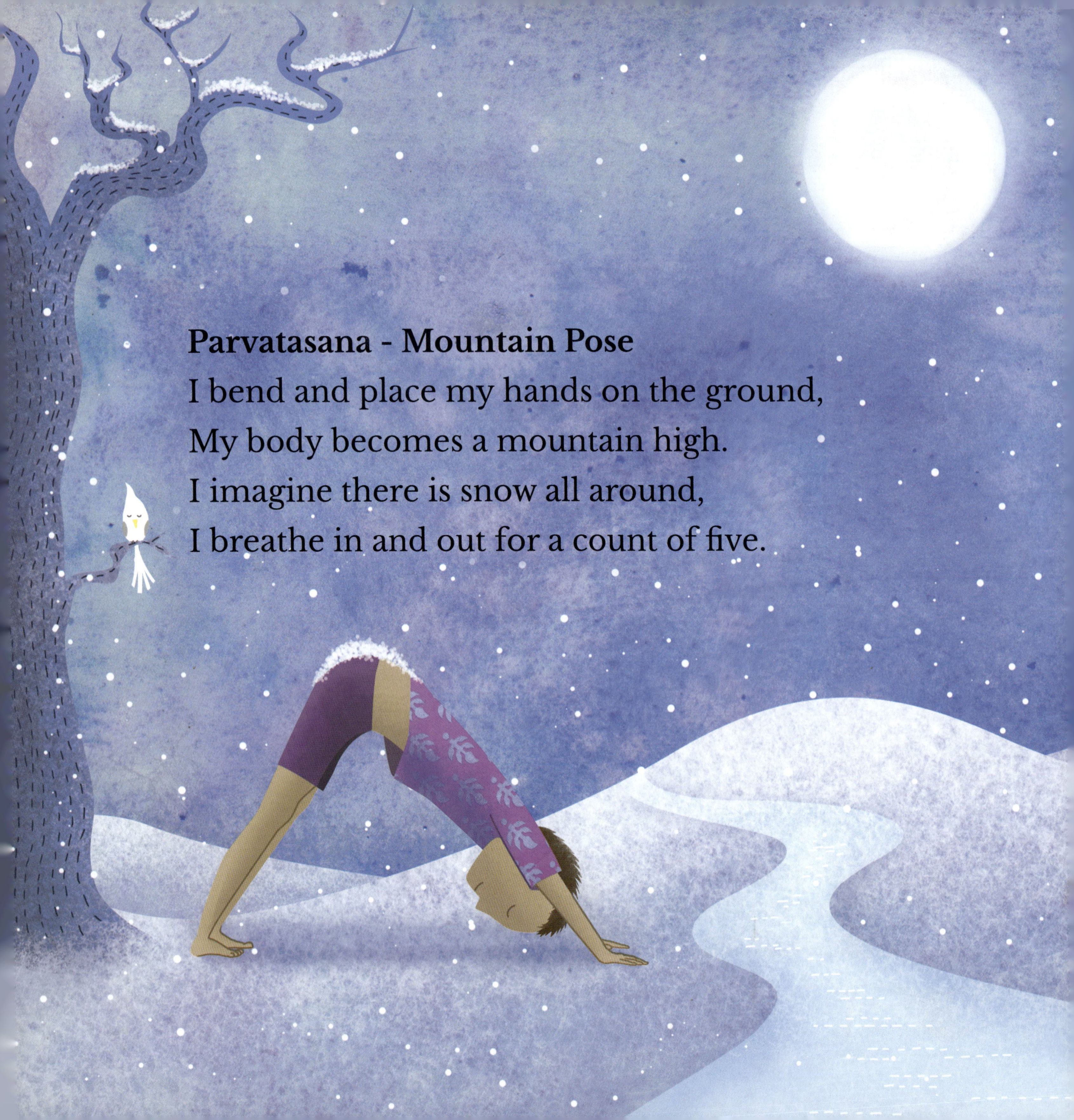

On me so many tall trees grow,
The pine, the fir, the walnut and oak.
Bushes adorn me and many streams flow,
In which the deer drink and sometimes soak.

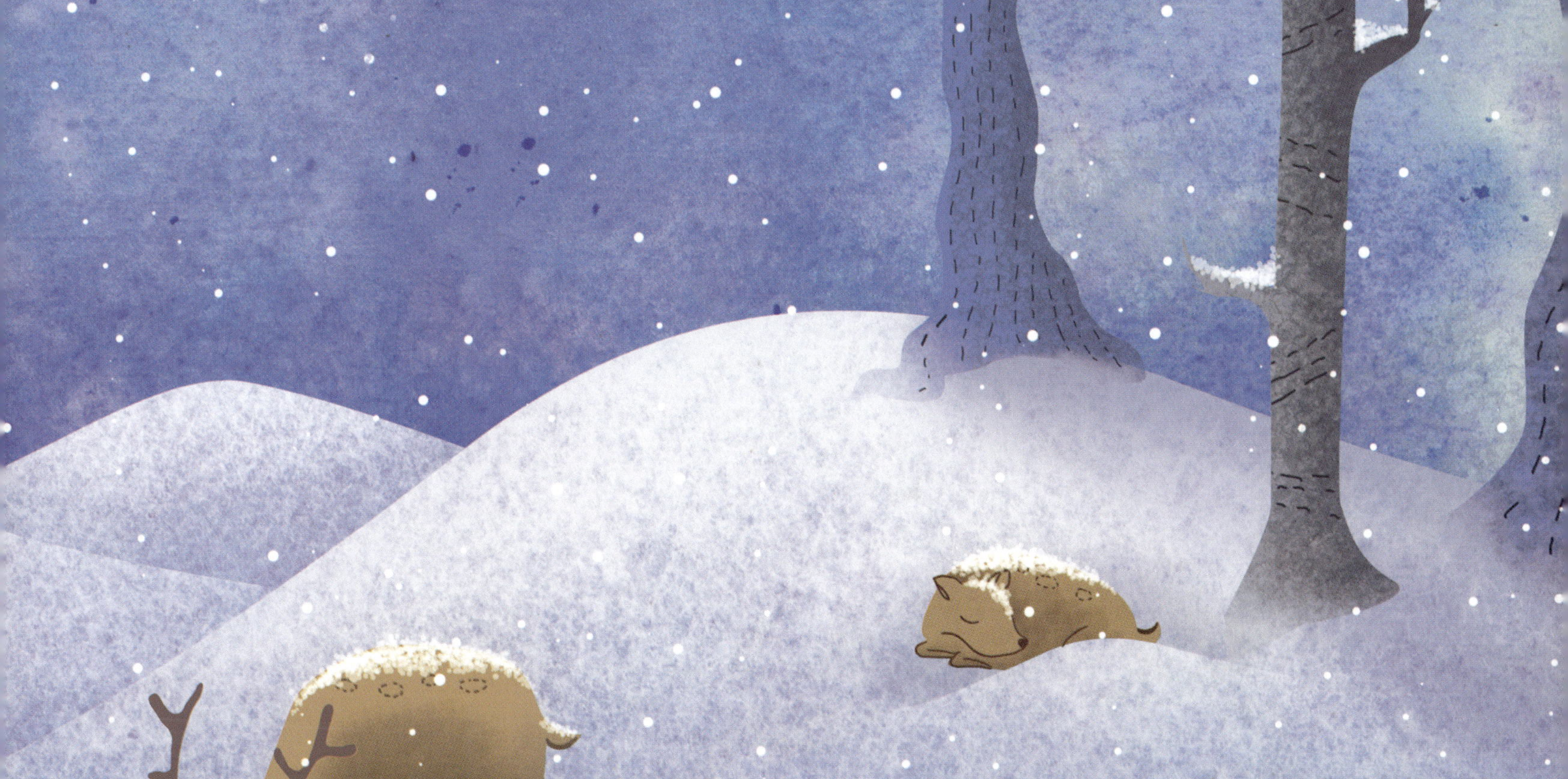

Strengthens arms, stretches the back and legs, stimulates blood circulation while developing the power of visualization.

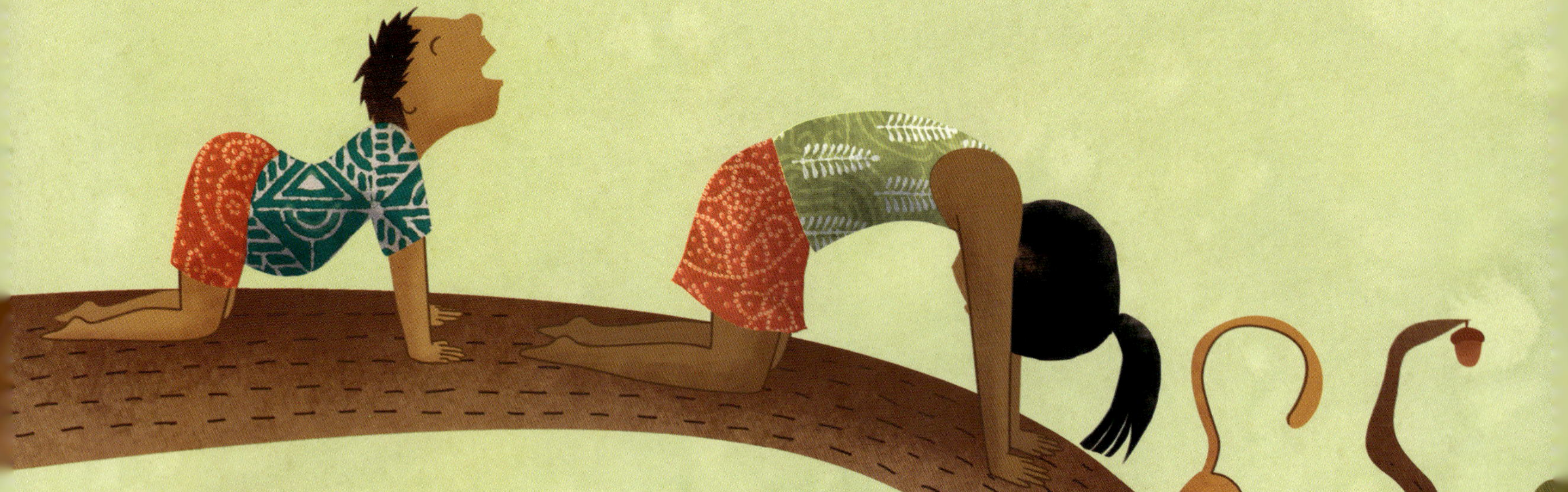

Marjari Asana - Cat Pose

I breathe in and arch my back,
Looking up I loudly meeoow!
Then breathing out I round my back,
Looking down, again I meeoow.

I do this five times, then, pleased with myself,
I decide to become a tiger instead.

Ensures a good posture, promotes mental and physical balance.

Vyaghrasana - Tiger Pose

Breathing in, I raise my leg and head,
Loudly I roar, all flee in dread.
Then down again and the second leg raised,
How powerful I feel, even I am amazed.

Five times with each leg, I'll be so strong,
Just like the tiger with its tail so long.
I can walk or run, race and jump,
Never do I give up, never do I slump.

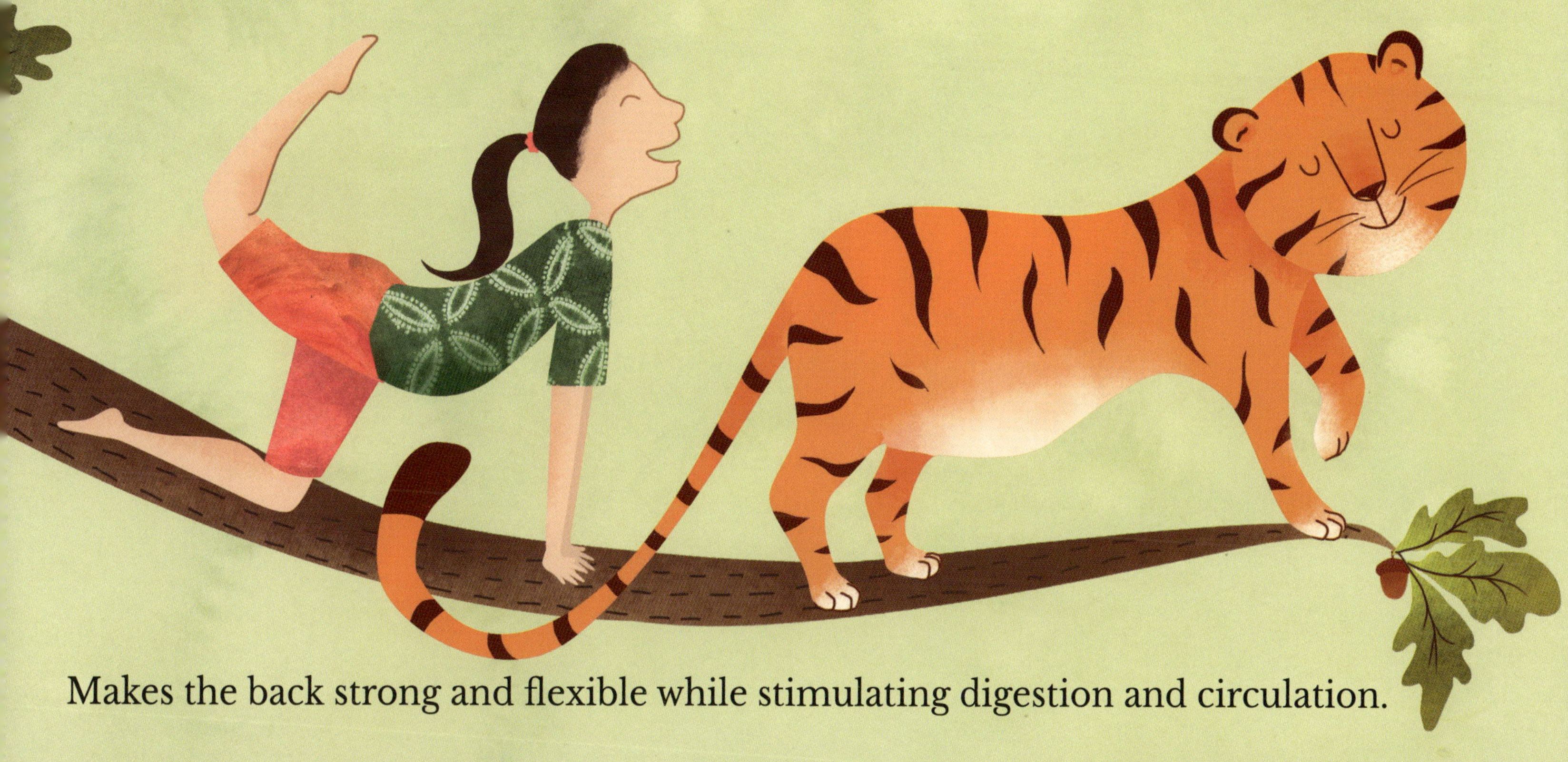

Makes the back strong and flexible while stimulating digestion and circulation.

Simhasana - Lion Pose

I am the king of the great jungle,
To me all bow, the proud and the humble.
Animals address me as "Your Majesty",
I either eat them or let them free.

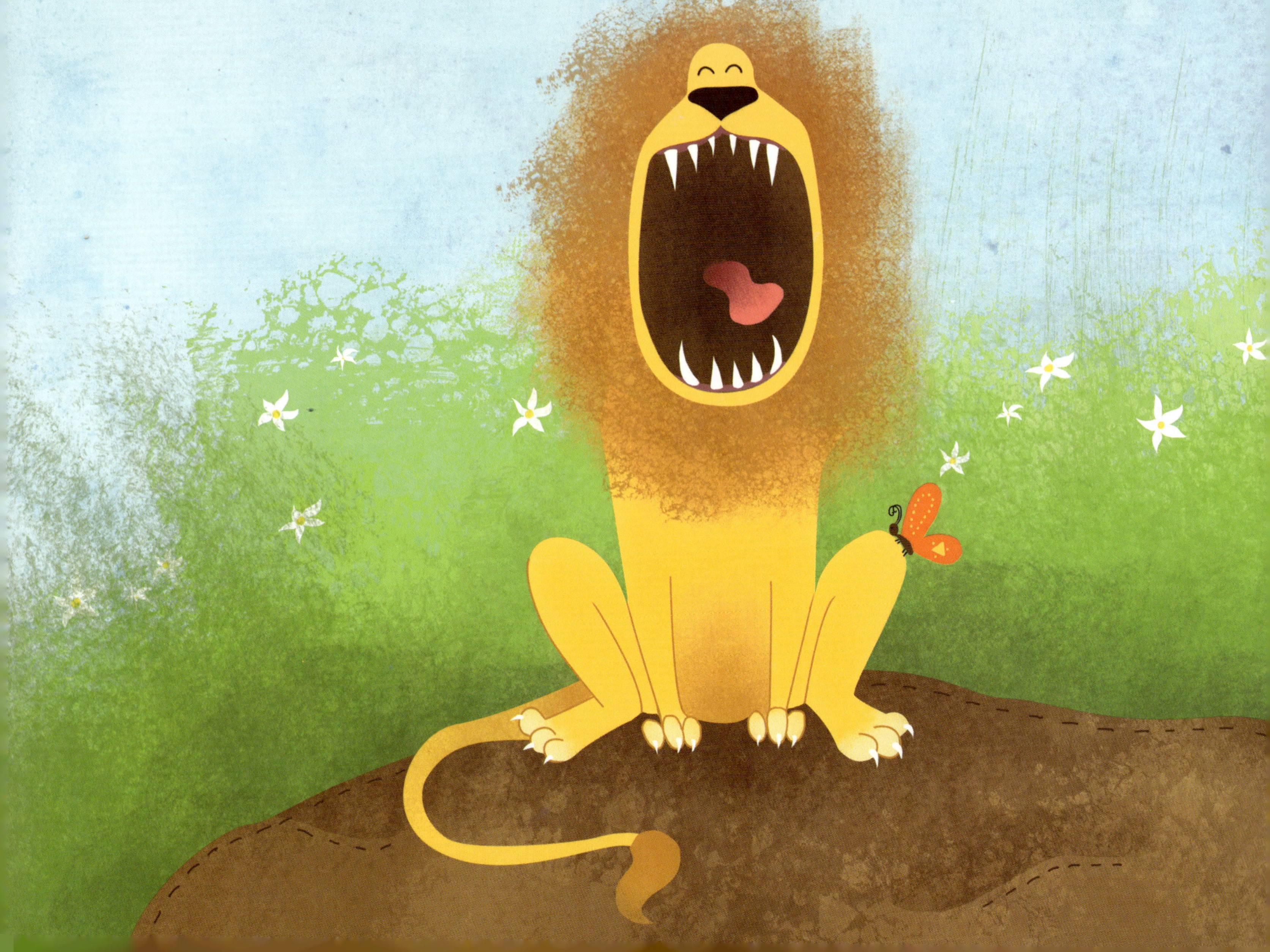

With head thrown back, inhaling through the nose,
I open my mouth wide and stick out my tongue.
While exhaling I roar ‘ahhhhh’, what a frightening pose,
Then I pause and repeat, and then I’m done.

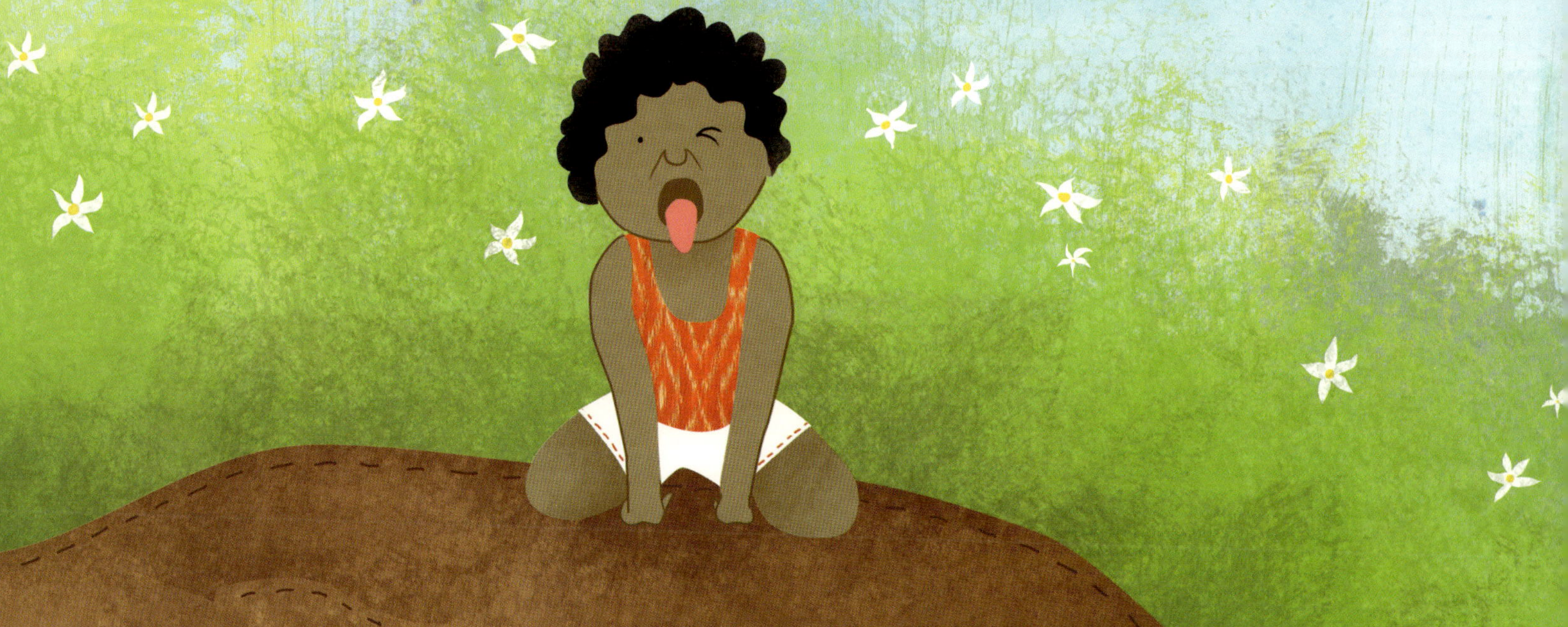

Develops a strong and beautiful voice, beneficial for those who are nervous and introverted.

Ushtrasana - Camel Pose

On my knees, I lift one arm,
Bending back, I catch my ankle.
I do the same with the other arm,
Catching with it the other ankle.

I am a camel who can stand,
The heat and cold of the desert sand.
I serve all people, young and old,
Who cross the desert, carrying their load.

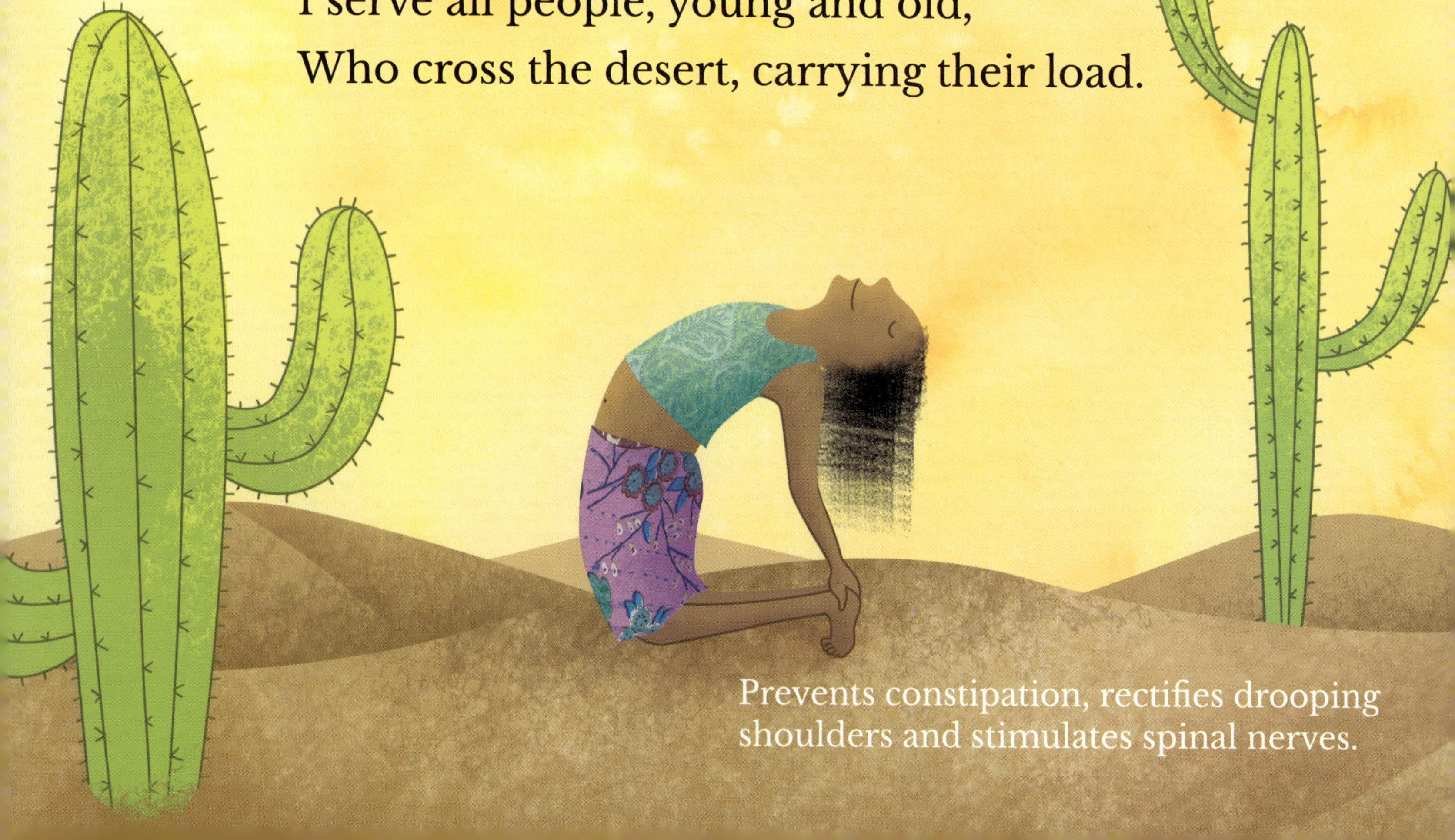

Prevents constipation, rectifies drooping shoulders and stimulates spinal nerves.

Balasana - Child's Pose

I place my head in front of my knees,
Curled up and comfortable, completely at ease.
I listen to my heart beating in my chest,
How hard it works, it never rests.

Thank you heart, for all you do,
I will also take care of you.
By eating all the right kinds of food,
That will make you strong and healthy, too.

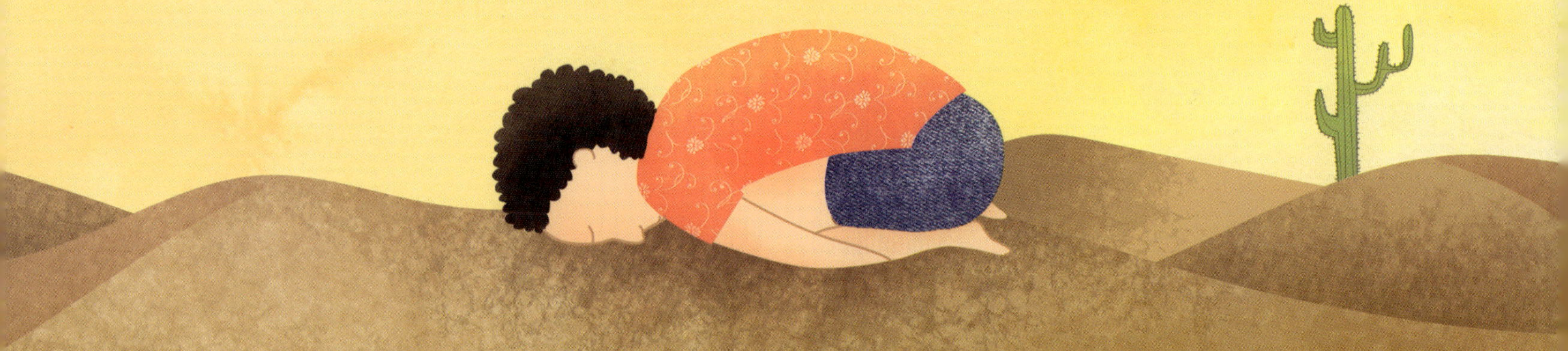

Soothes the nervous system, slows down heart rate and brings deep relaxation.

Shalabhasana - Flying Bird Pose (variation)
High up in the sky the little bird flies,
Over mountains, valleys and plains.
If only we could see through its eyes,
To it, all people appear just the same.

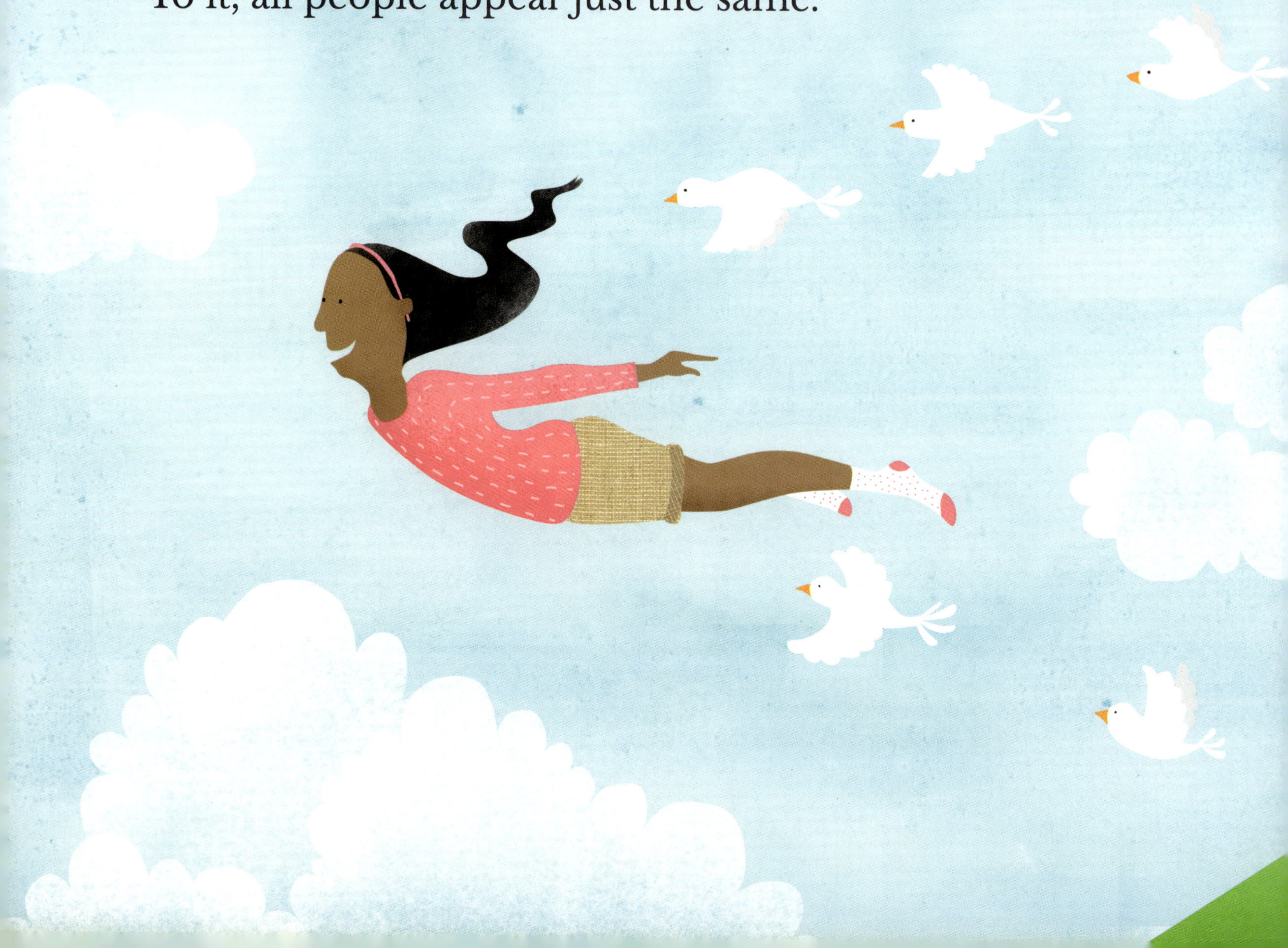

My arms and legs spread out like wings,
Inhaling I rise with a heart that sings.
Then exhaling I come down just a little bit,
Only to rise again, I simply love it.

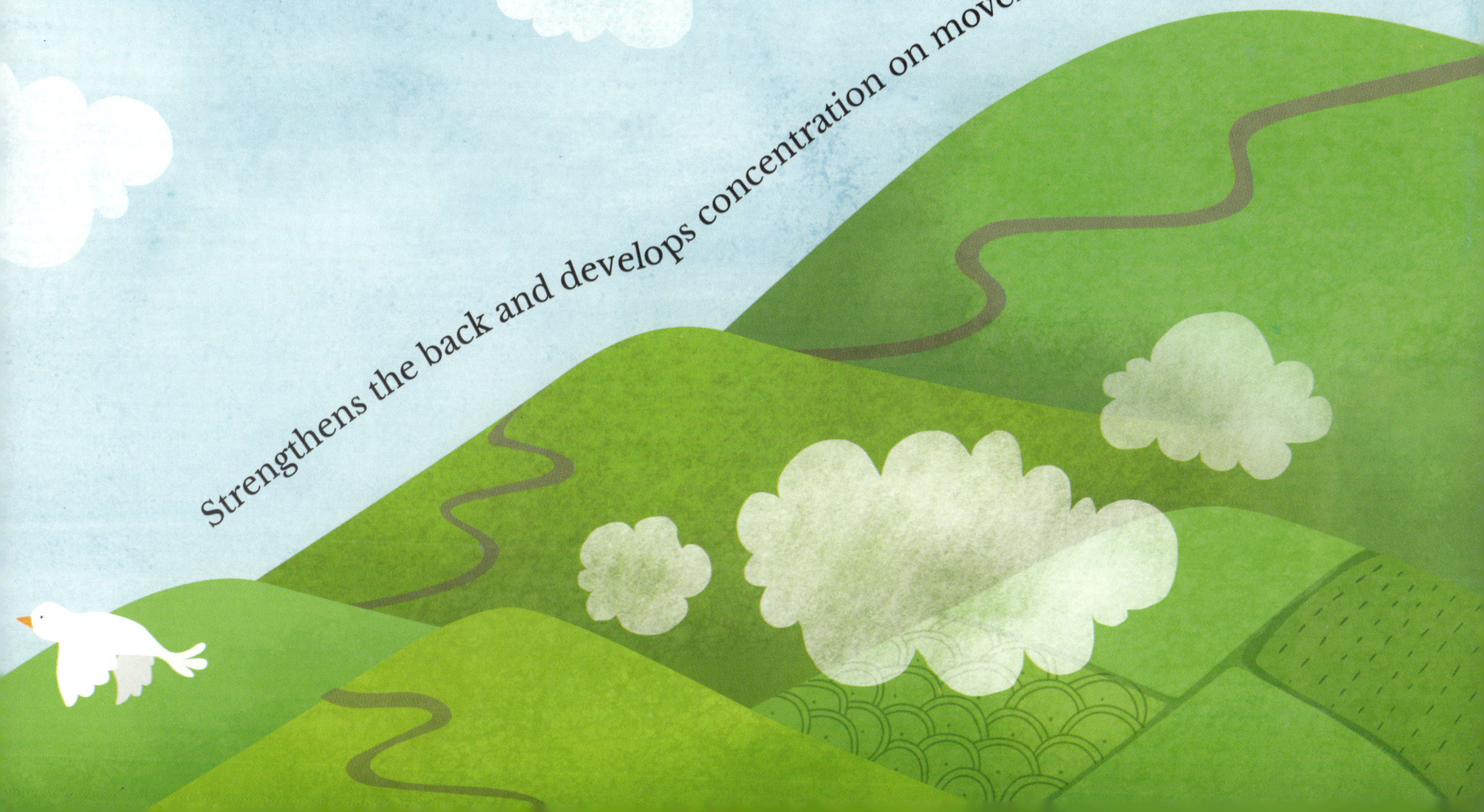

Strengthens the back and develops concentration on movement of breath.

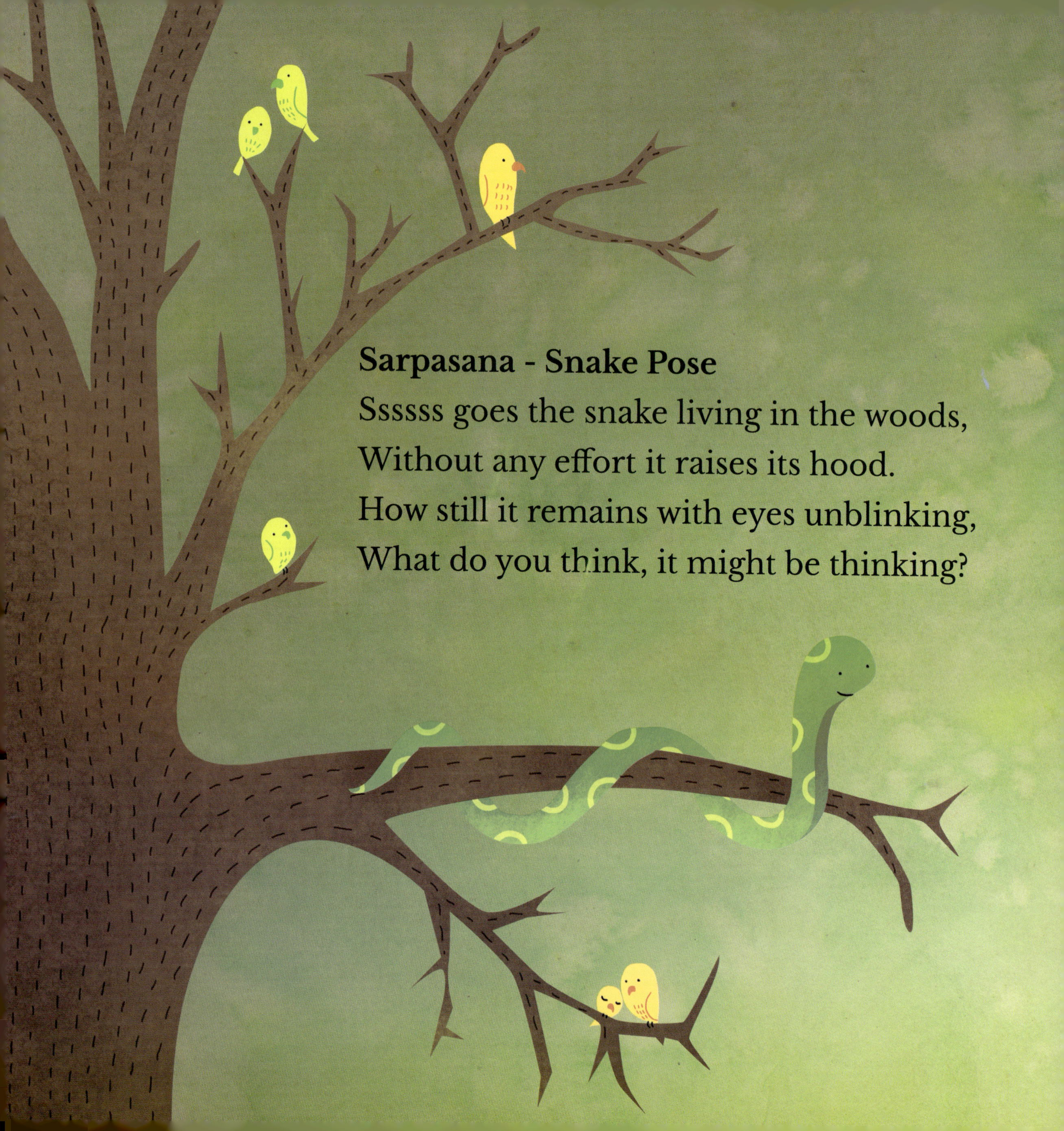

Sarpasana - Snake Pose

Ssssss goes the snake living in the woods,
Without any effort it raises its hood.
How still it remains with eyes unblinking,
What do you think, it might be thinking?

Tummy on the ground, forehead on the mat,
With fingers interlocked behind my back.
Three times inhaling, I raise head and chest,
And while exhaling, I come down and rest.

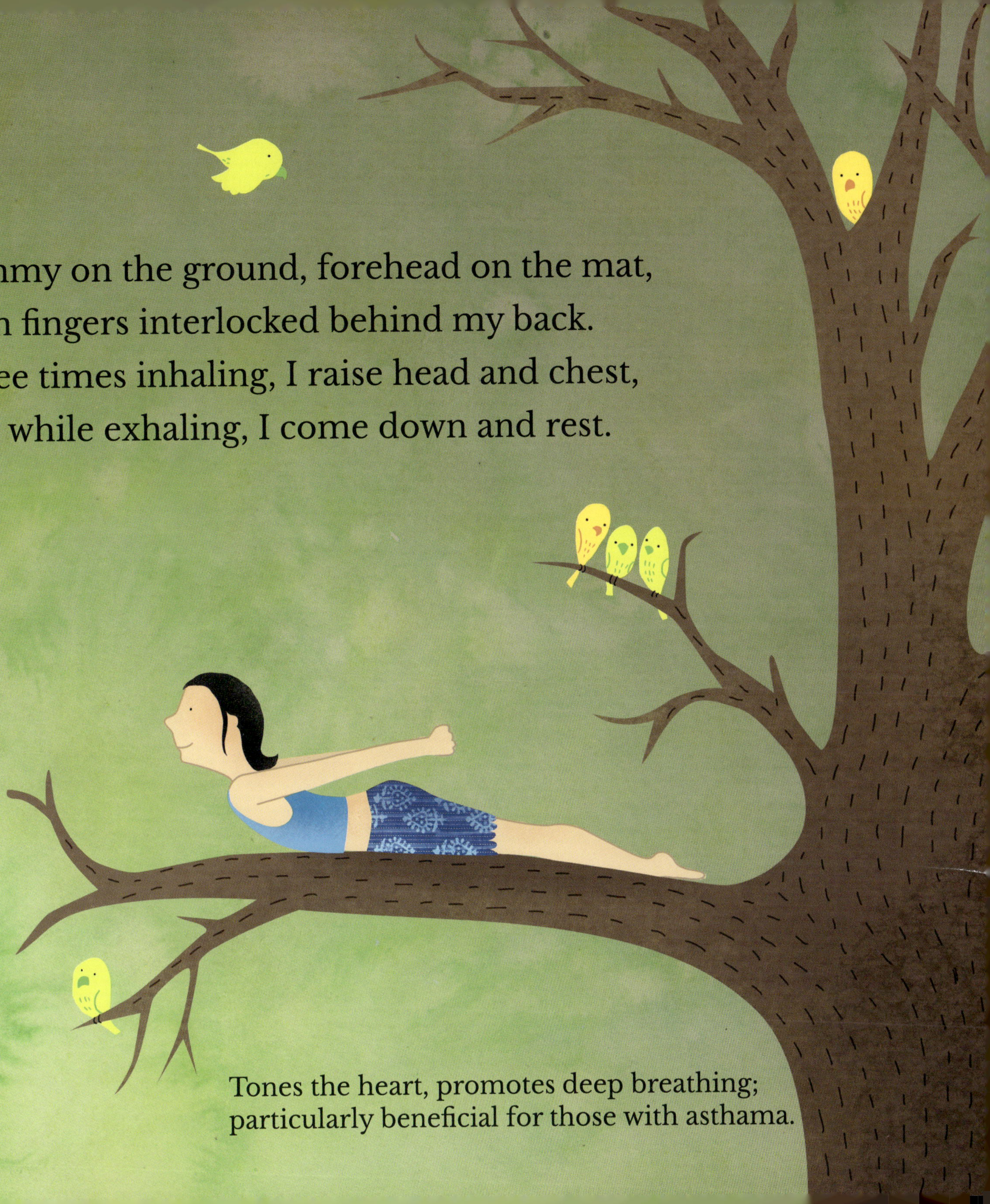

Tones the heart, promotes deep breathing;
particularly beneficial for those with asthama.

Makarasana - Crocodile Pose

I place my right hand on my left,
On that I place my head turned left.
And then I close my eyes and rest,
Of all the postures, I like this the best.

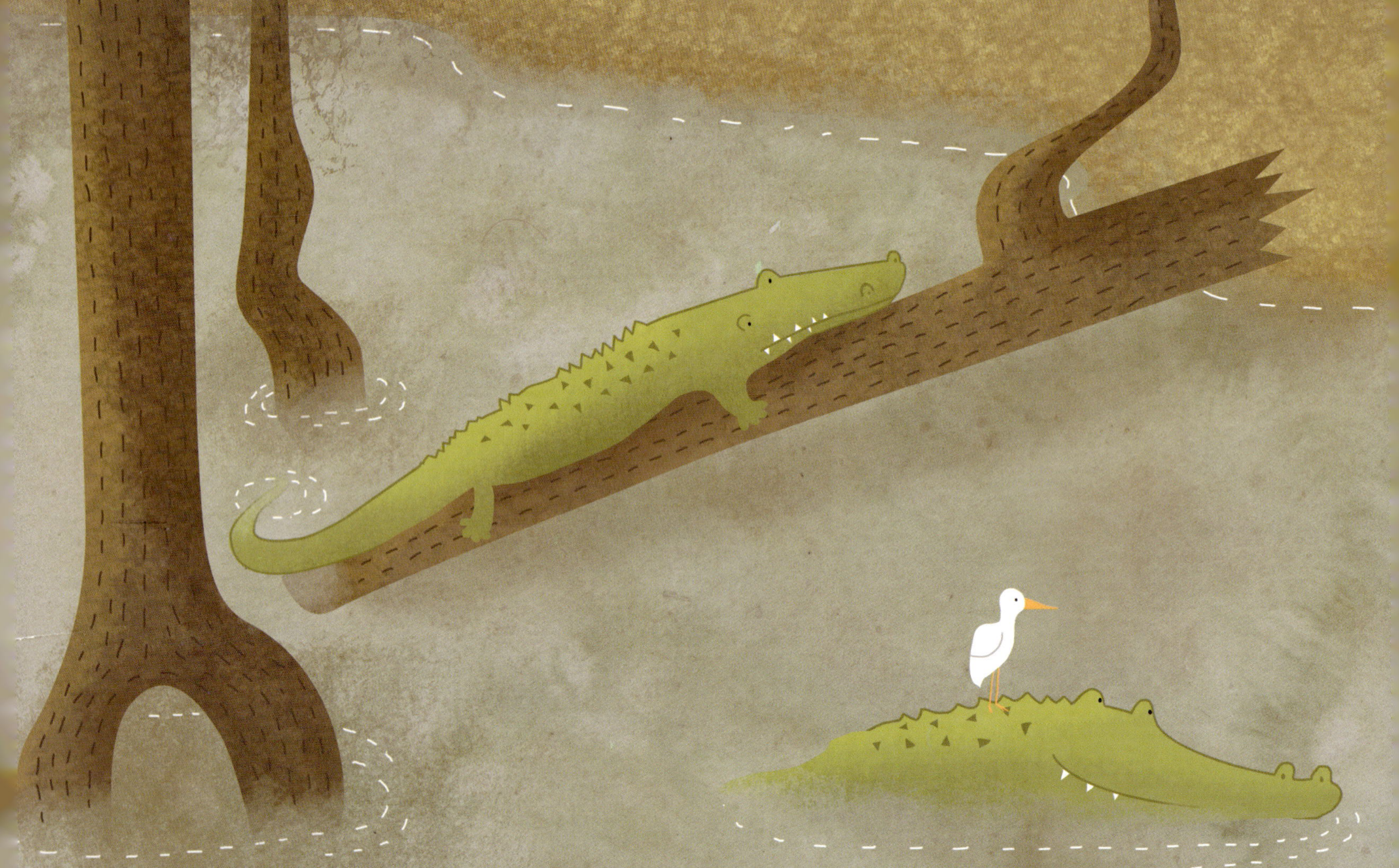

Relaxation is a state of full awareness of the breathing and the movement of the chest against the ground.

With chest to the ground, I deeply inhale,
Big toes touching, I slowly exhale.
Like a crocodile resting in the sun,
I remain motionless, it's so much fun.

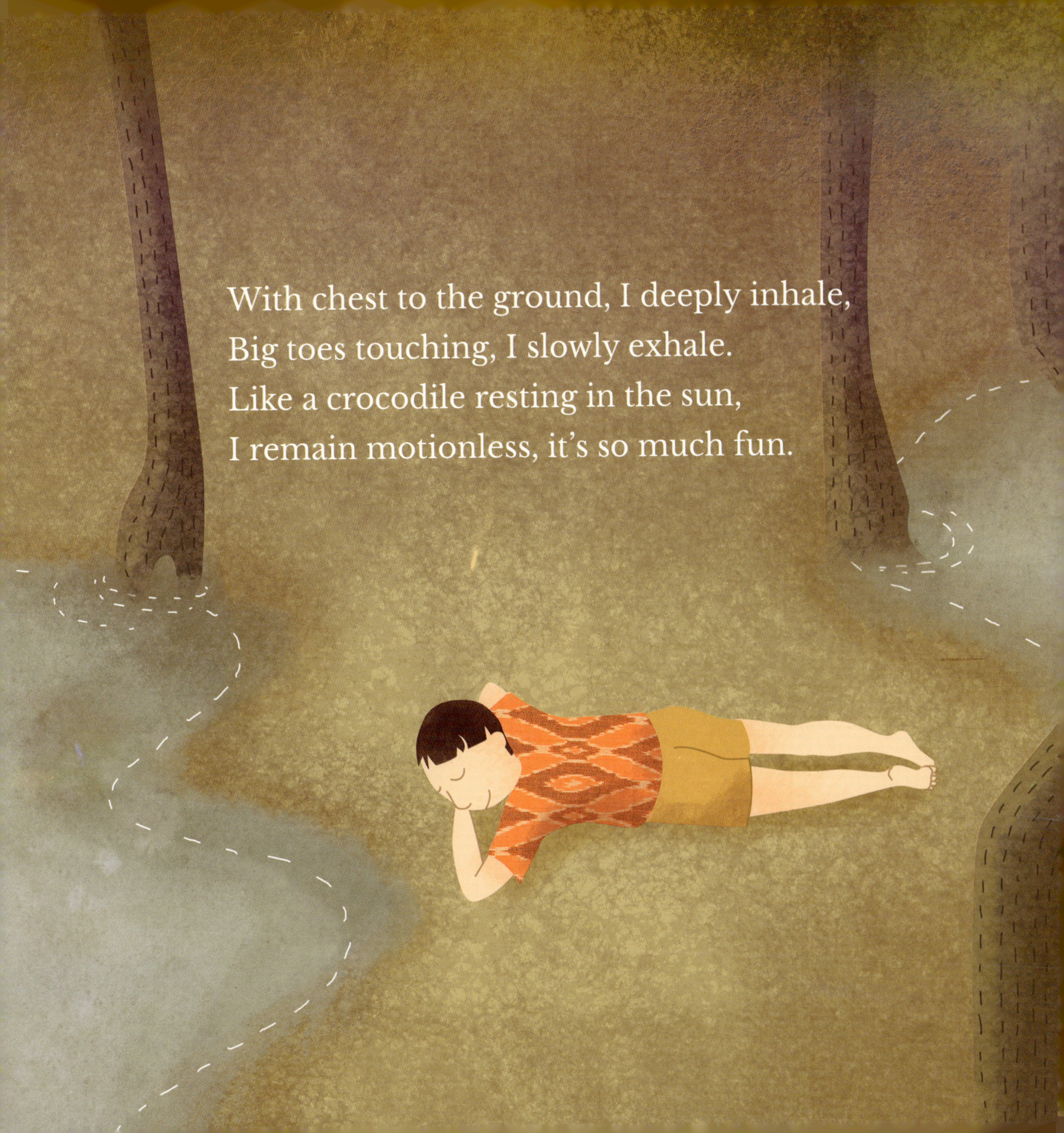

Sarvangasana - Shoulder Stand

I raise my legs up to the ceiling,
My body is straight, what a wonderful feeling.

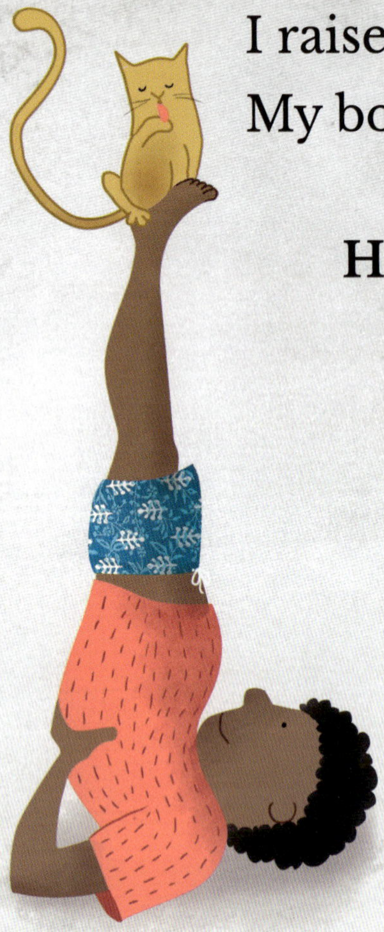

Halasana - Plough Pose

Then down come my legs behind my head,
My back will be strong and long, it is said.

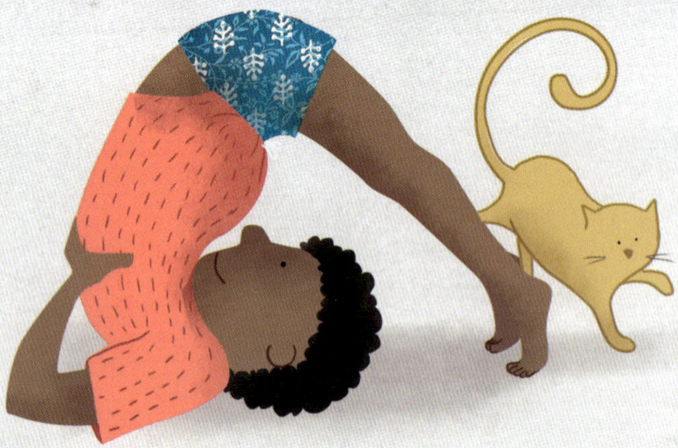

For a healthy thyroid gland and a strong immune and digestive system.

Setubandhasana - Bridge Pose

I catch my ankles and raise my hips,
Muffy the cat comes by and sniffs.
Under my bridge she slowly walks,
"Wow!" she would say, if she could talk.

Brings flexibility to the middle back and strengthens legs and wrists.

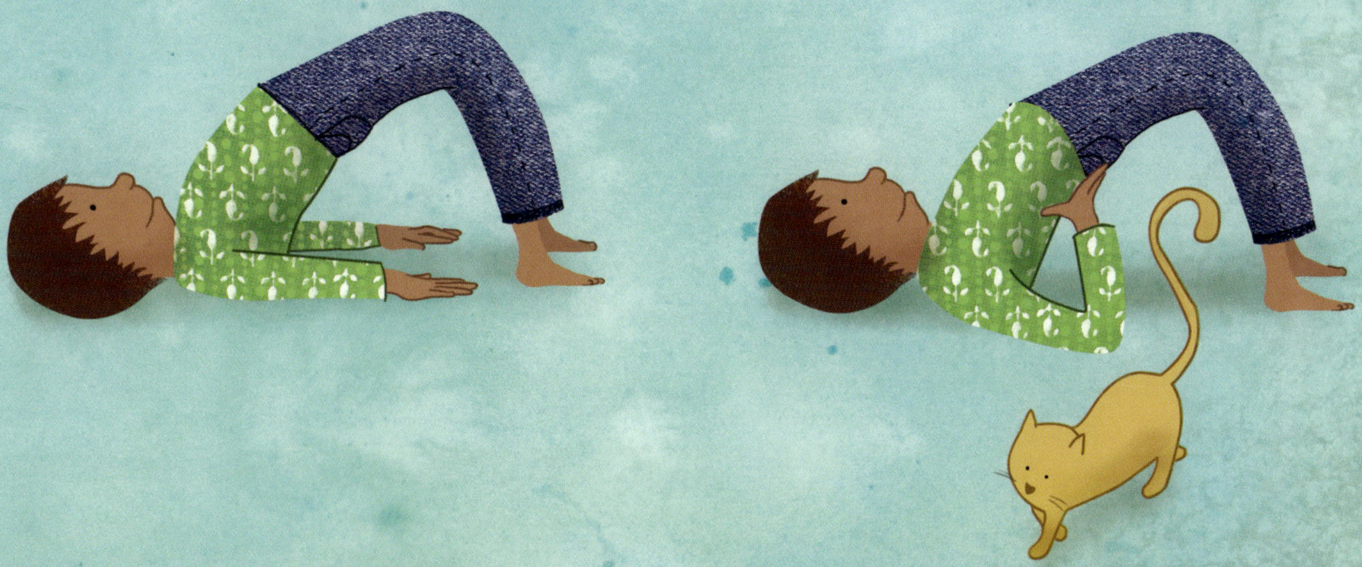

Matsyasana - Fish Pose

Arms together behind my back,
I raise my chest and drop my head back.
Like a fish floating in the lake,
Don't think I am sleeping, I am awake.

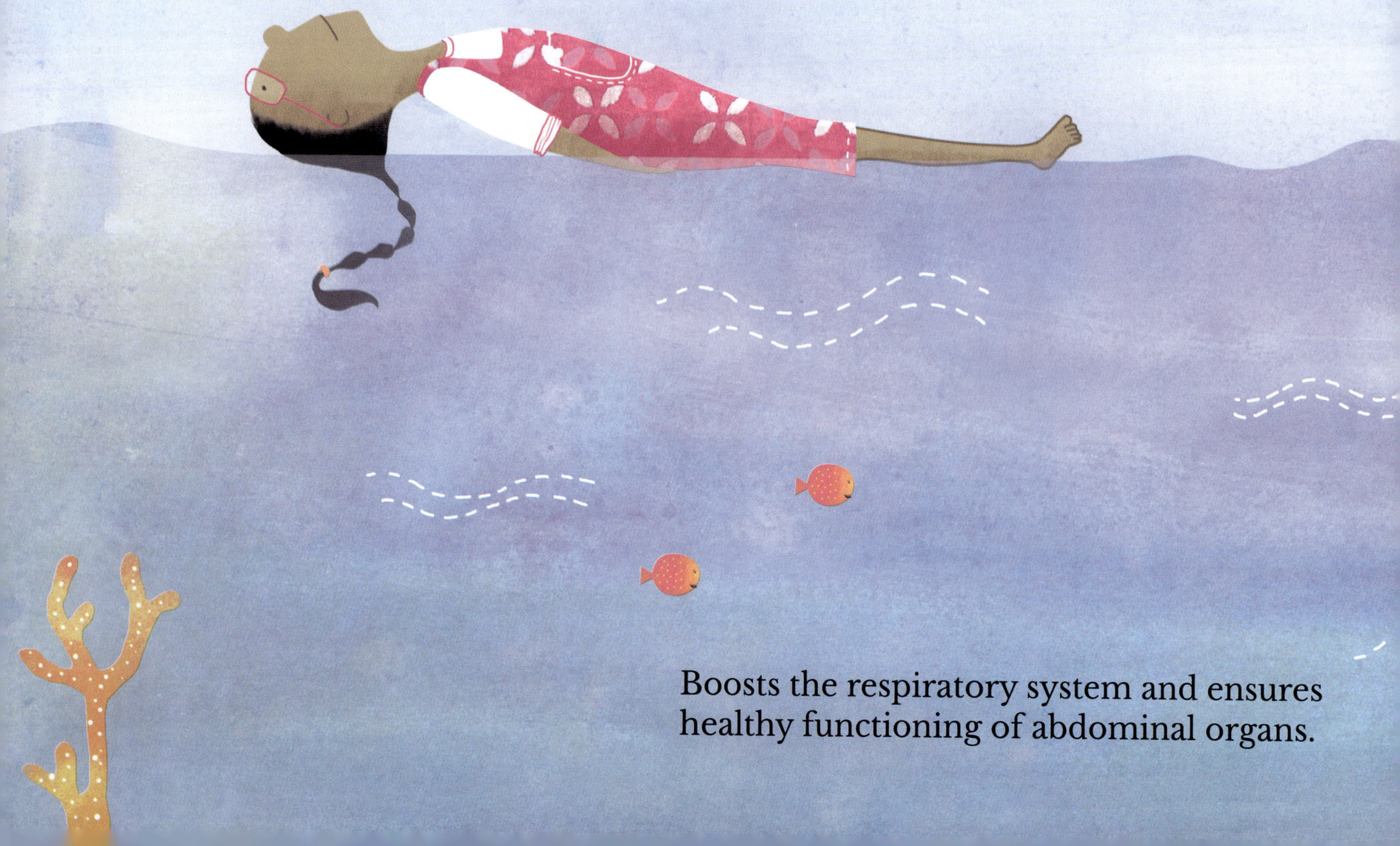

Boosts the respiratory system and ensures healthy functioning of abdominal organs.

Shavasana (again) - **Corpse Pose**
Now I close my eyes and rest,
My body is very nicely stretched.
I know it will be a beautiful day,
Thank you Yoga, for showing me the way.

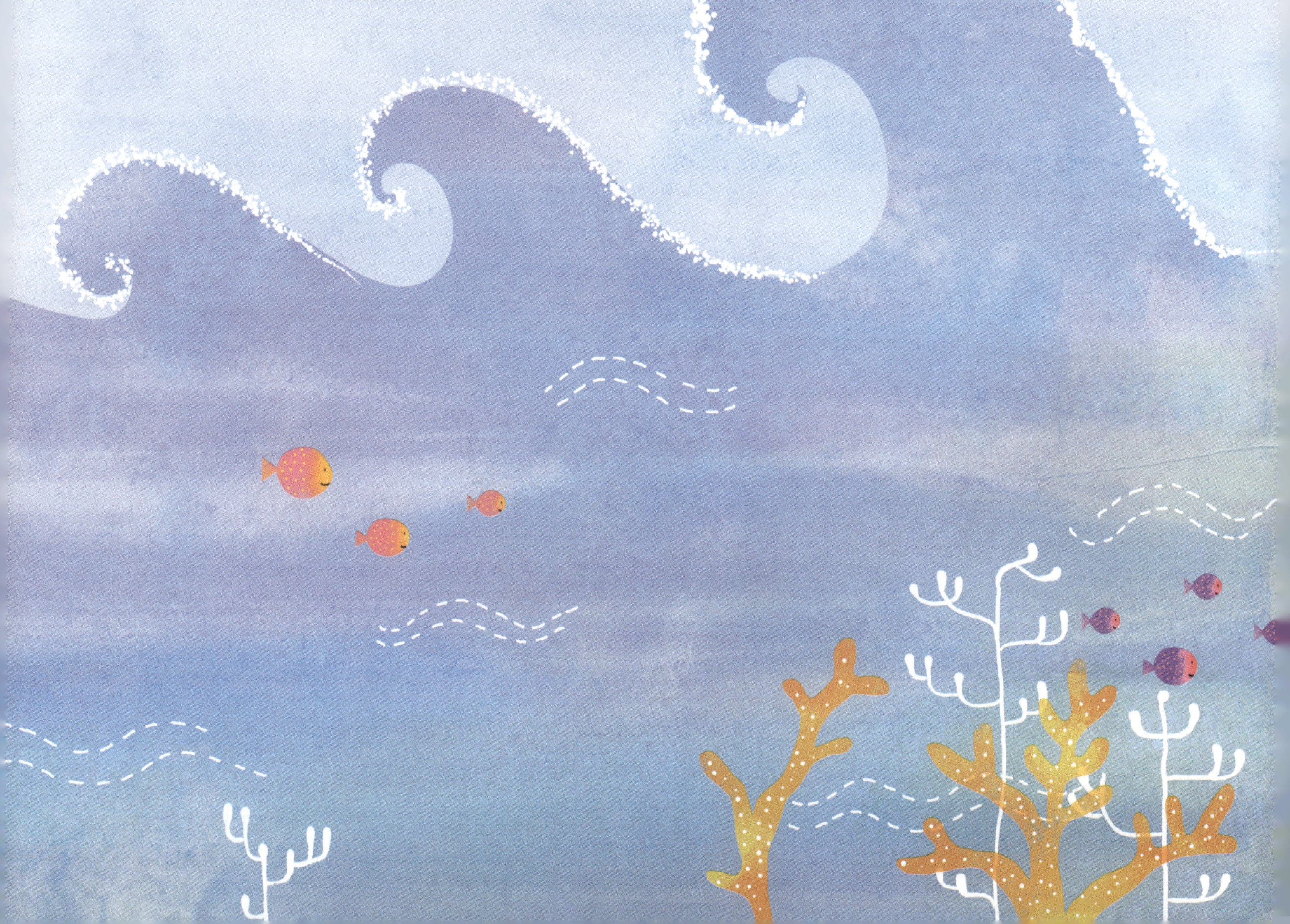

Padmasana - Lotus Pose

I am a lotus in the pond,
In silence do I grow and bloom.
I sit so still, no show, no shout,
Beautiful within and without.

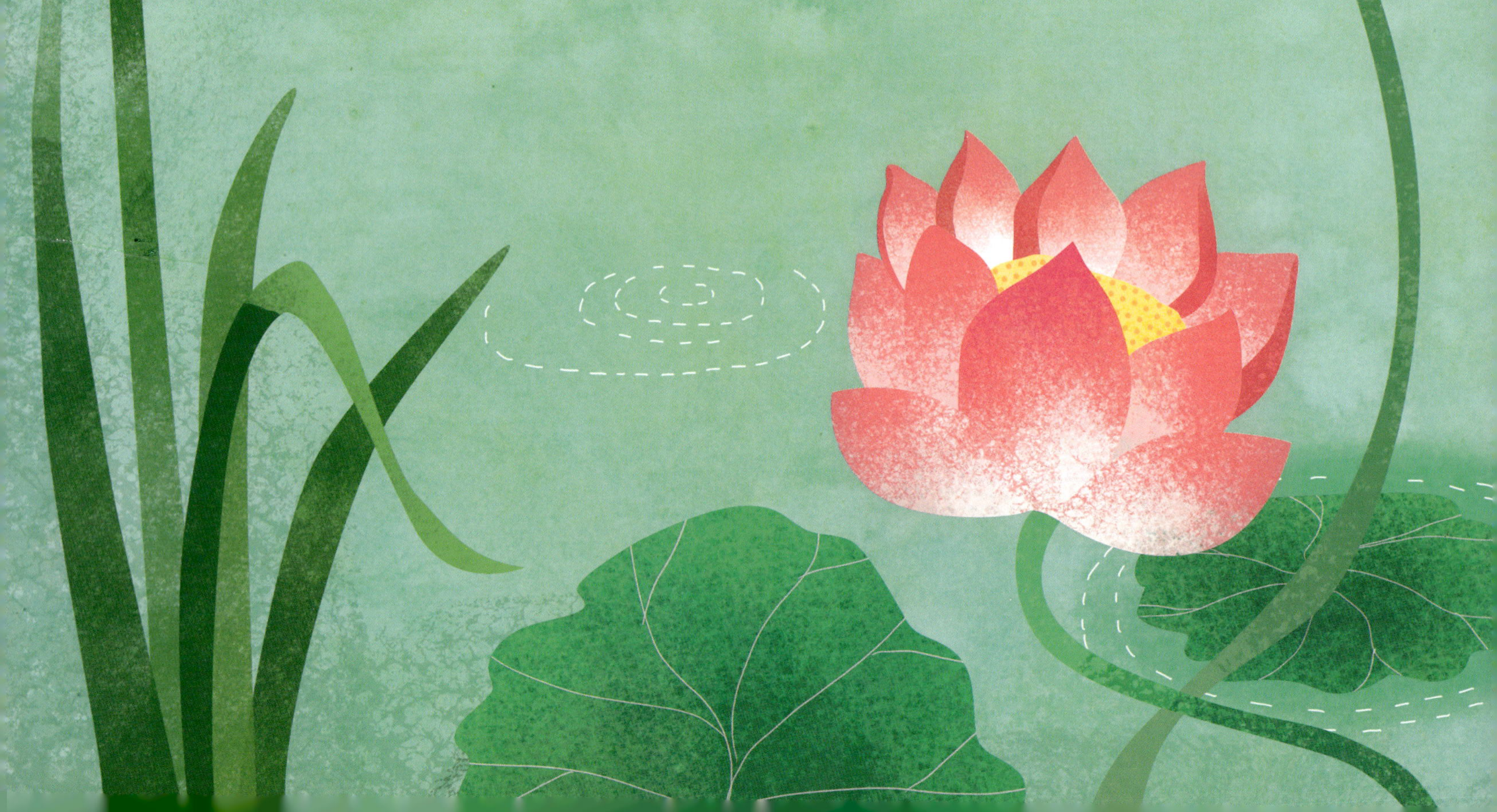

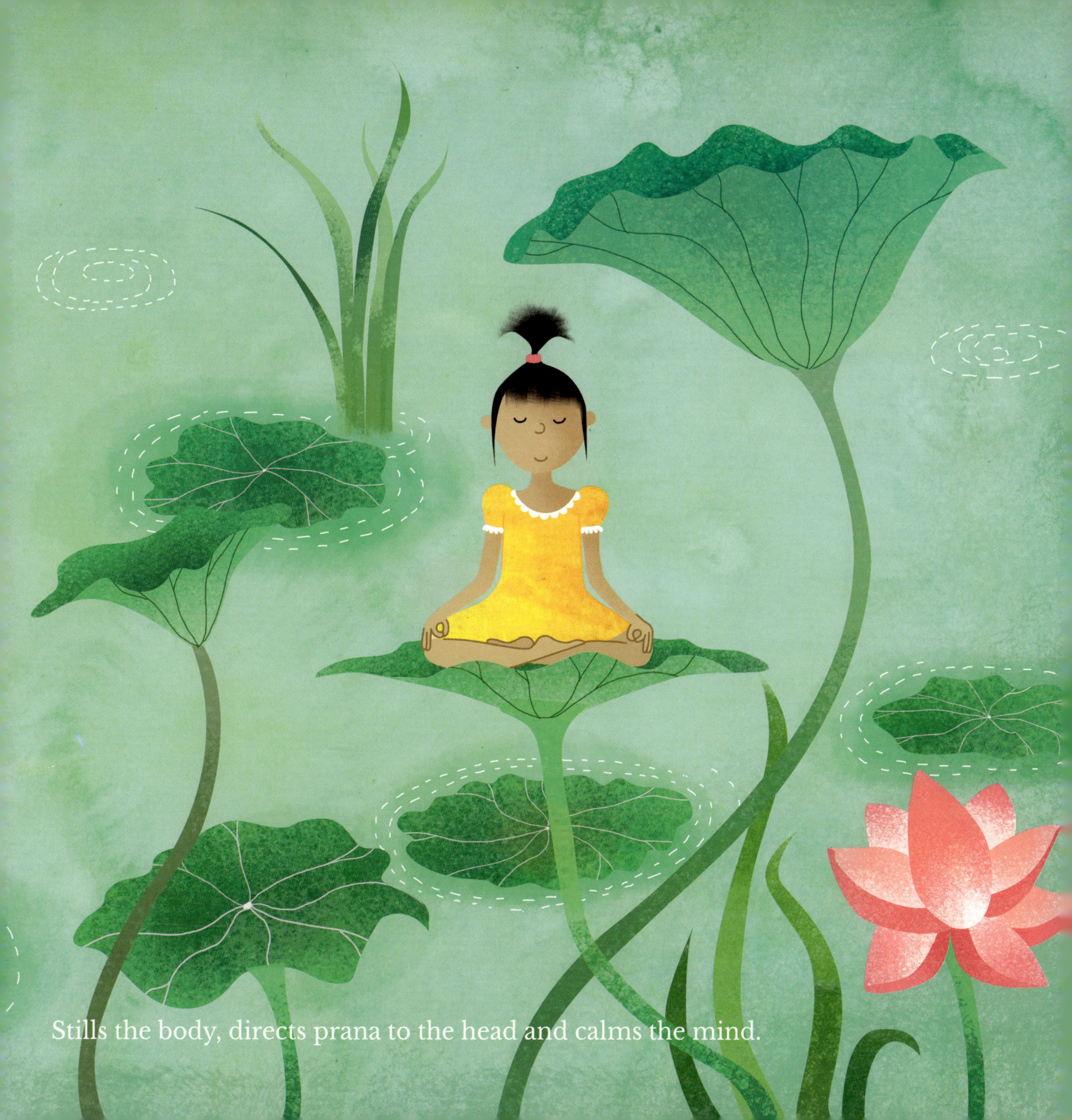

Stills the body, directs prana to the head and calms the mind.

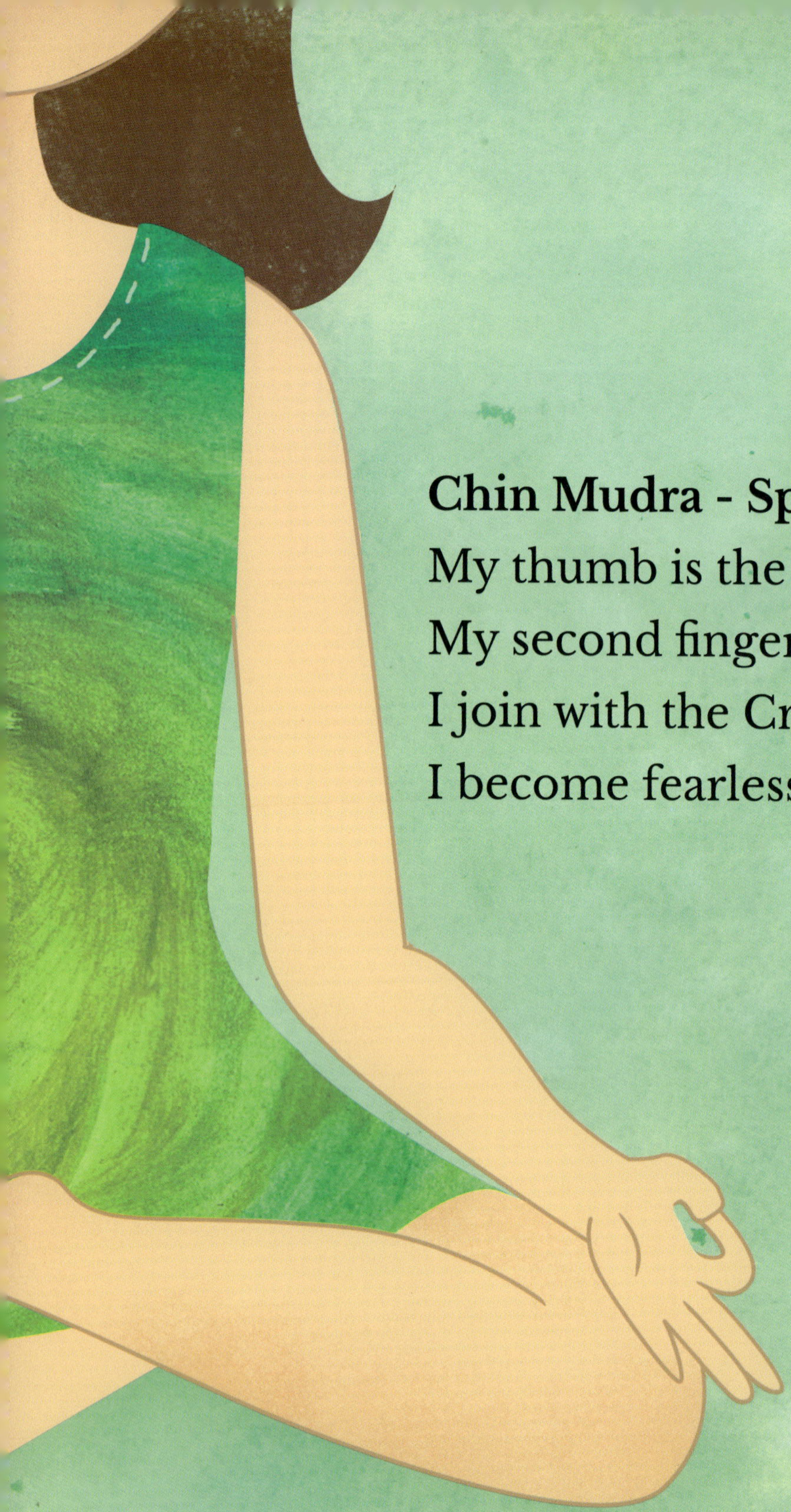

Chin Mudra - Special Hand Gesture

My thumb is the Creator who made the world,
My second finger is me, a part of this world.
I join with the Creator, then nothing goes wrong,
I become fearless, loving and oh so strong!

This finger-lock position makes the meditation asana more powerful.

Brahmari - The Humming Bee

Fingers in the ears and lips closed,
I breathe in deeply through the nose.
Then breathing out, I hum like a bee,
My head feels light, just try it and see.

I love the humming sound inside,
It makes me forget the world outside.
I enjoy sitting all alone,
In a beautiful world of my own.

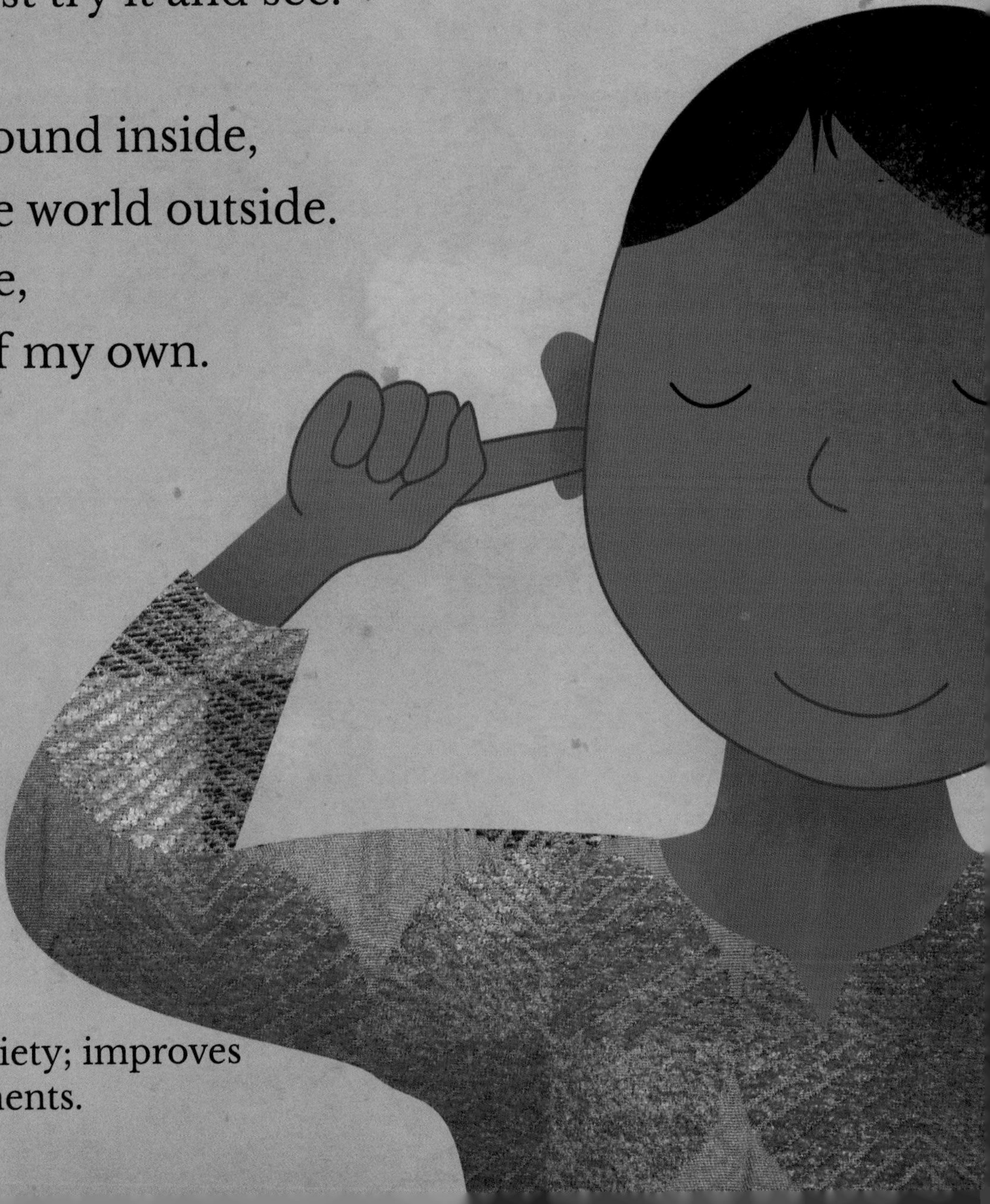

Relieves stress, anger and anxiety; improves voice and helps in throat ailments.

Deep breathing - Lying Down

I am the deep and mighty ocean,
In me the waves are in constant motion.
I breathe in and my tummy rises,
I breathe out and my tummy subsides.

Breathing in and breathing out,
This is what life is all about.
When the breath stops, I am no more,
So let me breathe right forevermore.

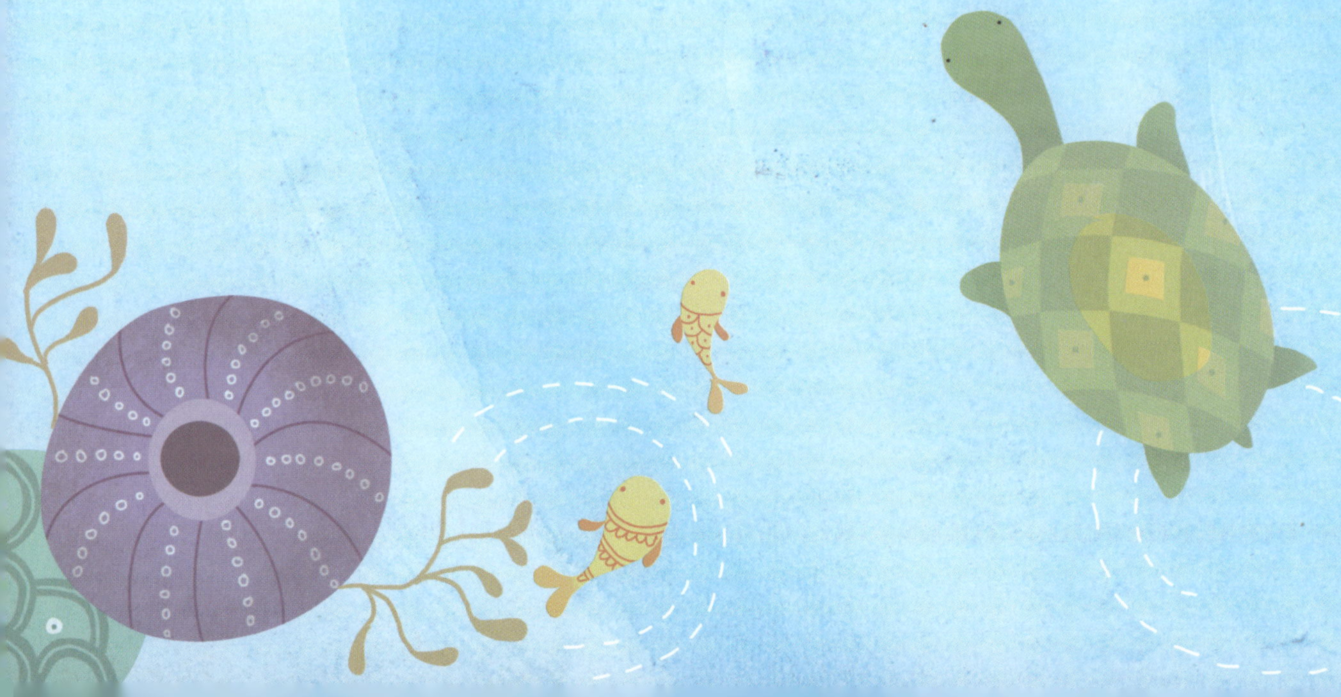

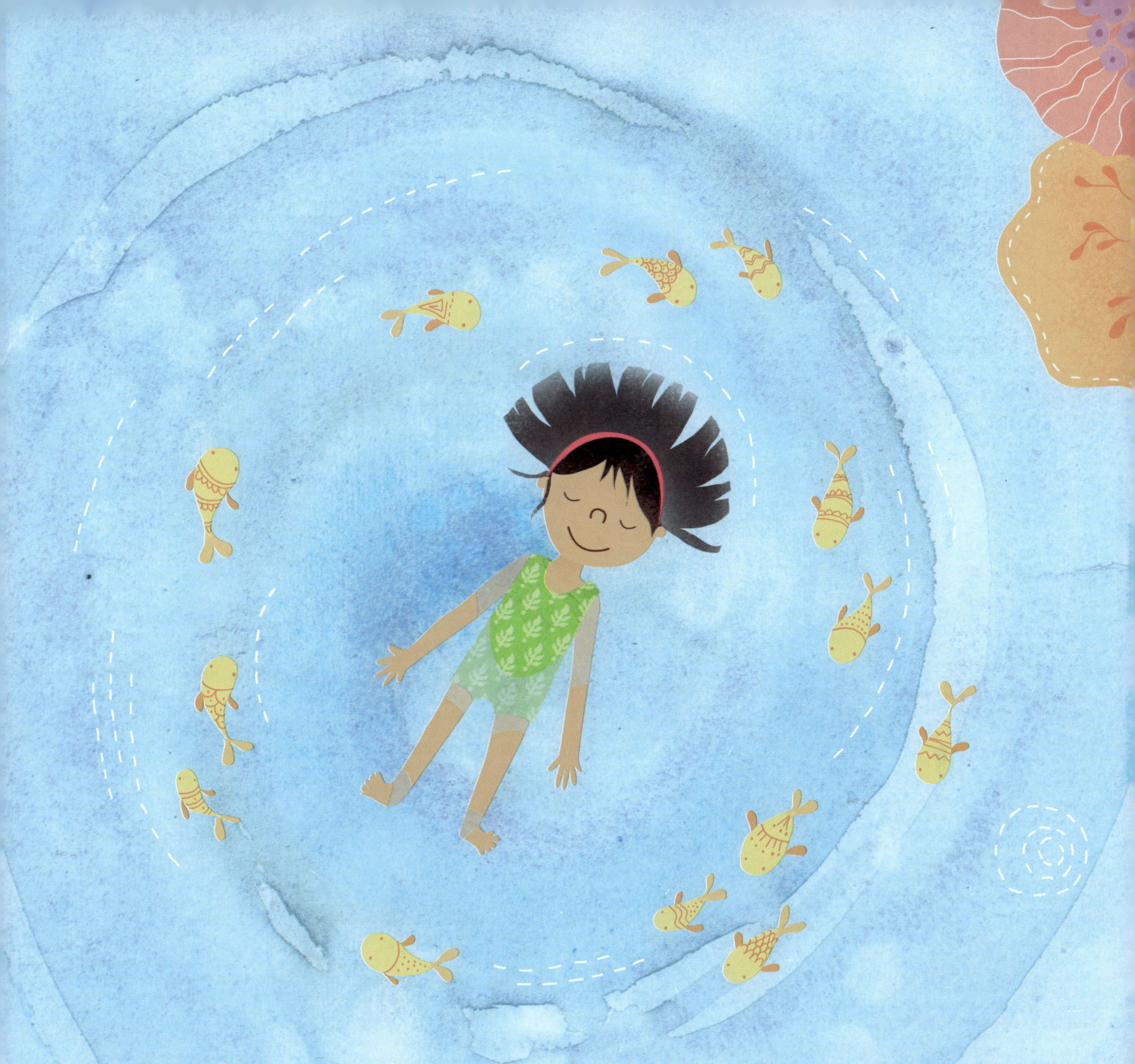

Observing the breath develops focus and results in a tranquil state of mind.

Meditation

In the morning I smile at the sun,
And open my petals, a new day has begun.
All around me other lotuses bloom,
They are white, pink, blue and maroon.

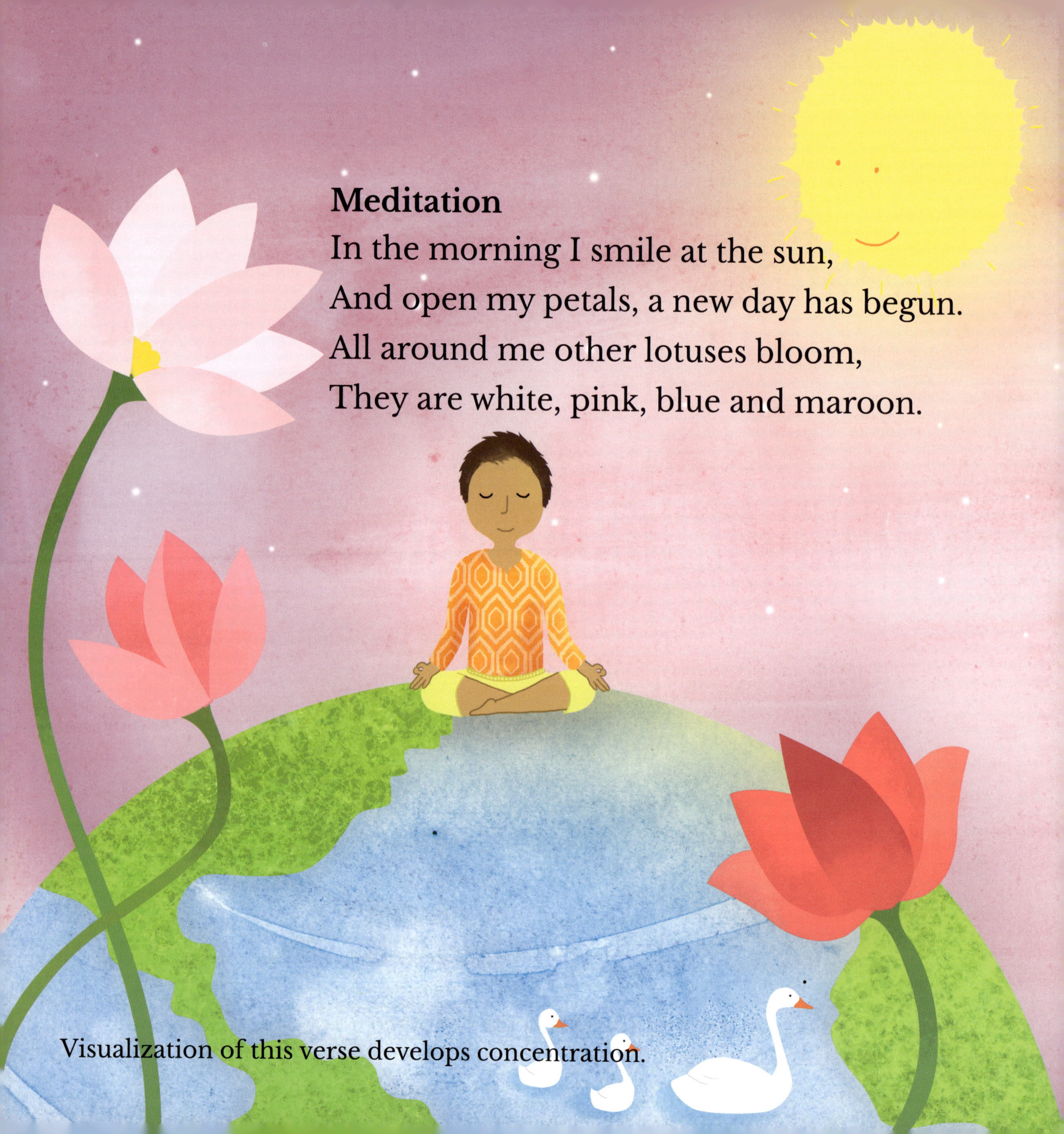

Visualization of this verse develops concentration.

With eyes closed I sit so still,
Nothing will disturb me, try if you will.
Deep in me I feel the thrill,
Of joy and peace, I have my fill.

The positive message to the mind in this verse deepens the silence and stillness within.

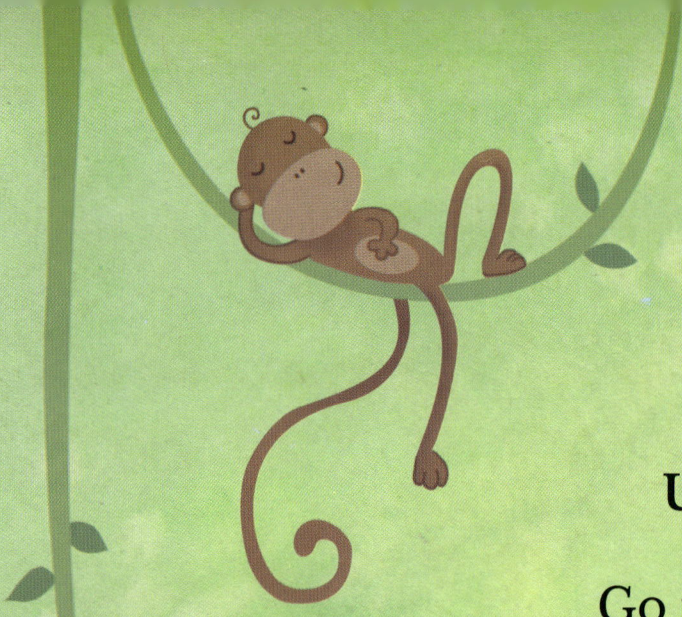

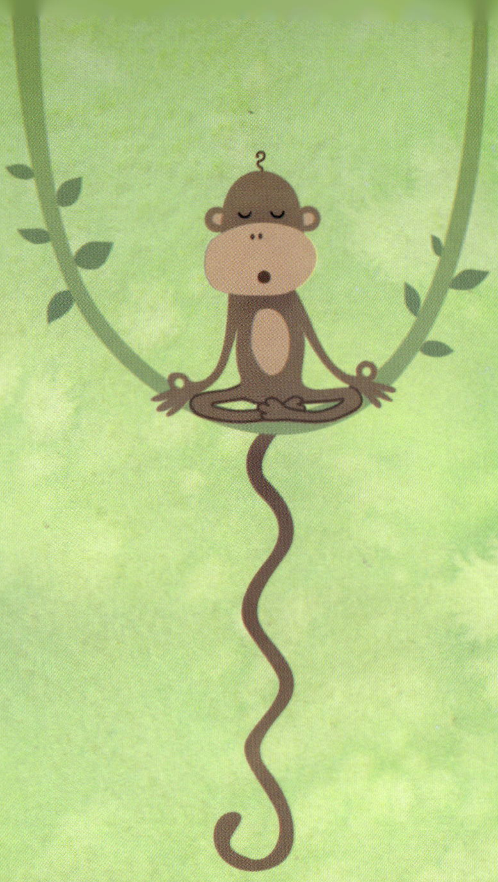

Useful Tips

Go to sleep early,
And wake up fresh.
Each day is new,
Don't be in a rush.

Eat lots of fruit,
Drink plenty of water.
Share your food,
With one another.

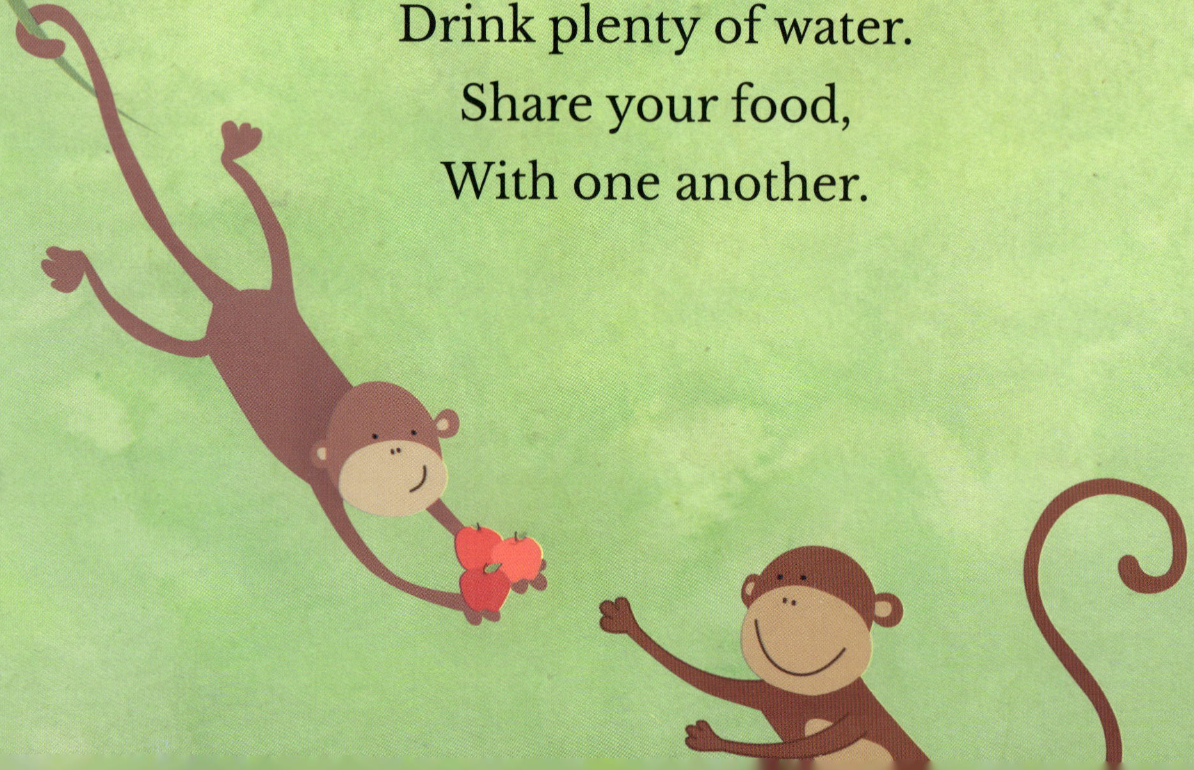